THE USER'S MANUAL FOR YOUR BODY

DR ANDREW RENAUT | Cancer Surgeon
& JOHN ARONIS

Creators of nysteia.com and the Nysteia Formula

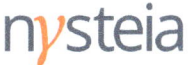

The User's Manual For Your Body

© Nysteia 2018

Published by Green Hill Publishing

First printed March 2019 by Lightning Source

All rights reserved. Except as permitted under the Australian Copyright Act 1968 (for example, a fair dealing for the purposes of study, research, criticism or review), no part of this book may be reproduced, stored in a retrieval system, communicated or transmitted in any form or by any means without prior written permission.

Title: The User's Manual For Your Body
Creators: Renaut, Andrew (author) and Aronis, John (author)
ISBN: 978-0-6484408-7-1
Subjects: Lifestyle, Health

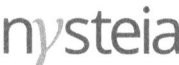

www.nysteia.com

Back cover icons from the Noun Project:
run by Samy Menai, diet by Nithinan Tatah

Dedicated to

Alyssa, Sophie, Anastasia and Illia

If we don't educate our children about the most important things in their lives – their health and their food – we needn't bother to educate them at all

THE AUTHORS

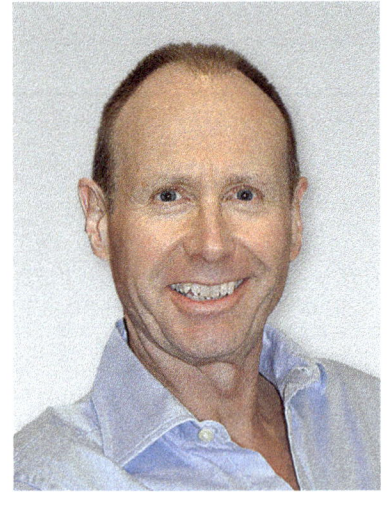

Dr Andrew Renaut
MS(Lond) FRCS(Gen) FRACS FDSRCS
Cancer Surgeon

Andrew is an Englishman who moved to Brisbane twenty years ago where he now lives with his two daughters Alyssa and Sophie, and where he runs a busy surgical practice looking after patients with cancer and other bowel-related conditions. He has spent forty years studying and operating on the human body and has a profound understanding of how it works particularly in relation to the food we put into it and what goes wrong when we feed it differently to how it has evolved. He is passionate about wellbeing and prevention and it's a constant source of disappointment seeing so many patients suffering serious disease and dying early because they haven't been given the right advice. With The User's Manual For Your Body he hopes to turn this around. He also has a master's degree in surgery for which he wrote a thesis based on some of the immune mechanisms in cancer. With this knowledge he has proposed the Renaut Hypothesis – he believes it is a defective immune system that causes many of the health problems, such as cancer, heart attacks, strokes and Alzheimer's, that are associated with obesity. When he's not doctoring, Andrew sails fast yachts, flies fast planes and drives fast cars. He also skis down mountains fast and is an accomplished chef; he likes doing all of these things in the company of his two daughters. He maintains peak physical and mental fitness by using the Nysteia Formula every day.

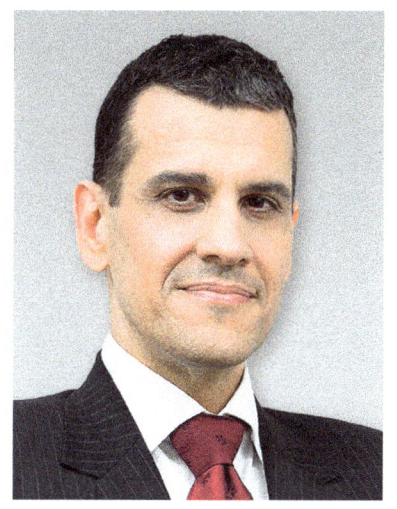

John Aronis
BBus(Acc) GradDipCA MCom MA

John was born in Sydney, and raised in Brisbane where he lives and pursues his broad range of interests. He has a bachelor's degree in business, a master's degree in commerce, and a master of arts in political and international studies. He is a chartered accountant and chartered tax advisor, and is principal of his accountancy business based in Brisbane. John experienced a personal battle with obesity for many years, and like many individuals was left frustrated and totally confused by the lack of information on how best to deal with it. After studying the topic extensively and putting into practice the Nysteia Formula he has now reached his biological optimum weight (BOW). And importantly, he will never again become overweight and progress to obesity. When he is not working, John likes to maintain his physical and mental wellbeing by continuing with the Nysteia Formula on a daily basis. He is a trained classical guitarist, and enjoys flying planes, walking in rainforests, and practicing the Japanese martial art of Aikido.

Disclaimer

The content of this book is general advice only and mostly represents the personal views of the authors. Under no circumstances should it be used as personal medical advice. If you have concerns about your health you should seek the assistance of a qualified health professional.

CONTENTS

	Introduction	viii
1	How your body digests and uses food	1
2	The food that you eat	20
3	How your body stores excess food	32
4	Insulin and why insulin resistance is so critical	39
5	The real meaning of metabolism, health and fitness	58
6	Why physical activity & exercise are essential	62
7	How your body fights disease and illness	66
8	The diseases that are even more common in obesity	71
9	Why you will get sick and die early if you have obesity	86
10	What your ultimate goal should be	89
11	The Nysteia Formula – the three things you need to do to change your life	93
	Appendix	98
	Abbreviations and their definitions	100
	FAQ	102

INTRODUCTION

Why you need The User's Manual For Your Body – The purpose of a user's manual – What are Nysteia and the Nysteia Formula? – How to use The User's Manual For Your Body

Why you need The User's Manual For Your Body

Mankind is sleep-walking into the biggest health disaster in the history of the World – on a scale far greater than any plague, pestilence or famine that we have witnessed previously. All of the advances we have made in modern healthcare will be completely negated by it. We are of course referring to obesity and the increased risk of disease that goes with it. This is no longer conjecture – the statistics and our personal experiences support it. We have been collecting data on morbidity and mortality for many decades now, and have seen a steady rise in both improved health and lifespan, as a result of increased sanitation and medicines that have cured contagious illnesses. By comparison, advances in the treatment of heart disease and cancer for instance have been relatively modest, but they have nevertheless all contributed.

That upward trend, in certain age groups, is already slowing down and will almost certainly plateau and then continue into a decline. It is the tip of the iceberg because many of the conditions we're talking about are chronic and have a long lead-time. In twenty years we will look back and ask ourselves "where did it all go so wrong?" – by which time it will be too late. The overwhelming irony is that all of this is largely preventable and mostly reversible. The fact that we're not preventing and reversing it leads to the inevitable conclusion that most people simply don't know how their body works.

So YES – you definitely need **The User's Manual For Your Body.**

The purpose of a user's manual

Whenever you buy anything new, of a vaguely technical nature, whether online or in a store, it comes with a user's manual. This applies to obvious things like a car, a sound system for the home or a washing machine; but you also get one for simple toys and games for example. It's usually in the form of a pamphlet but sometimes, depending on the complexity of the product, it extends to a little booklet and very occasionally a veritable tome. Most products now don't actually come with a hard copy – the information is available online.

Luckily most of the things around you are designed to function intuitively i.e. you don't need to think too hard about how to put it together or how it works. And that's because manufacturers realised a long time ago that impetuousness and laziness are innate human traits, so if it isn't obvious how something works then you won't buy it.

Most of the time you don't read the user's manual which makes it obsolete – it goes straight from the packaging into the trash can, still in its plastic wrapper. But manufacturers still issue them with the vain hope that one day you might actually get around to reading it, but mainly so they can protect themselves in the event that the product suddenly stops working. At the very least they can turn around and say: "well if you'd just followed the instructions we wouldn't be having this conversation".

But even if you can work out things intuitively it's probably to your benefit to still read it thoroughly. Firstly, there will be a few things you didn't realise it could do and so you often don't take full advantage of its usefulness; and secondly, for it to function optimally, there's a few things you need to do along the way – in a car it's called servicing – and this also ensures longevity.

The more valuable something is, the more careful we tend to be at looking after it so that we get the most out of it and in particular making sure it lasts as long as possible. We are probably more likely to read the user's manual and in particular the servicing schedule.

But here's the most astonishing bit of irony: the one thing that you should cherish more than anything else – no exceptions – is your own body. Yet when you arrived in the World you didn't come with a user's manual. And here is something equally astonishing: nobody has ever written one for you, so that you might make maximum use of it and importantly ensure that you last a long time and, for the majority of that time, go about your daily life without any worries.

Bizarrely, we do a very good job at trying to destroy it; and as for servicing – forget it! The really good thing though is that the human body has simply wonderful powers of in-built servicing and repair so that, however hard we thrash it, there will be an attempt to bring it back to optimal function. This process is called homeostasis. But there is a limit to what it can take as you will discover later in the book. If you push it in this direction hard enough it sure as hell will go wrong and often irreversibly.

What are Nysteia and the Nysteia Formula?

The User's Manual For Your Body is an add-on to Nysteia - a website that we have developed over the past couple of years. Nysteia's philosophy is about allowing you to lead a happy, healthy longer life through using the Nysteia Formula. Nysteia is so called because it is ancient Greek for fasting – they were the first people to appreciate the benefits of fasting, not for obesity necessarily but more to sharpen the brain, one of the other many benefits.

It is not another fad diet – it is a method of eating and living, based upon the science of the human body and in particular how it handles the food you put into it. It's actually very simple and involves three things: **intermittent fasting, cardiovascular exercise and Mediterranean-type cuisine**. Doing just one or two of the three in isolation will almost certainly not allow you to reach your BOF (biological optimum function) and BOW (biological optimum weight). To understand why this works and, in reality, why it is the *only* thing that works, you must have a basic understanding of the human body and food and how the two interact. And that's exactly what this book gives you.

How to use The User's Manual For Your Body

There have been countless books written about the human body – in particular how it's put together, how it functions and the diseases that affect it. They are mainly written by doctors for doctors as an aid to their training. But as far as we know there is nothing that constitutes an actual "User's Manual" for the everyday person. A book that tells you how things work in a way that you can understand and importantly containing vital information about the food we eat.

This user's manual is not a book just about food or nutrition or diseases. It's pretty much the same as a user's manual for anything else. It gives you some basic understanding of how the body is put together, how the various parts work, how to keep it running smoothly, how to prevent it from going wrong, and how to keep it going for its intended life. For this particular product there isn't a service schedule because, by and large, it fixes itself – but only if you allow it to!

The book has eleven chapters and, in this respect, it can be used as a reference manual; but it has in fact been written to be read like a novel from cover to cover. It goes into some basic human anatomy, in particular the gut, and how it deals with the food we put into it. It includes information on the way we have evolved, how we stay on an even keel, how we digest our food, the way the body stores food, and autophagy which is the body's own way of dealing with potentially harmful cells.

It then covers the types of food we eat and what happens to them once they are in the body. We then dedicate quite a lot of space to the role of insulin and the development of insulin resistance, and make no apology for doing so – it is a hormone and process that are absolutely key to what causes obesity. It introduces the new idea that insulin resistance, considered by many to be a disease, is in fact a normal survival mechanism that has evolved to help us conserve our energy substrates. It also explains the idea that, when taken beyond its intended role, insulin resistance affects our immune system, allowing us to become sick.

We then go into the concepts of health, fitness and metabolism – terms that are used often without people really understanding their true meaning. This is followed by a chapter on physical activity and the importance of exercise. We've dedicated a whole chapter to the immune system because, once again, it is something that is poorly understood but is absolutely critical in determining our health. This is followed by a section on some of the diseases and illnesses that are more common in people who have obesity. Finally, we introduce the concepts of biological optimum function (BOF) and biological optimum weight (BOW) and how these should be your ultimate aim, by getting back insulin sensitivity. A brief, but significant, chapter is dedicated to the Renaut Paradigm which explains how insulin resistance potentially affects our immune system, leading to serious disease and early death.

The very final chapter is entitled The Nysteia Formula. In effect this is the quick-start guide. If you're not that fussed about reading the whole book, that's fine – we won't be offended. But if you want to know how to get started here and now then you'll find it in this section. We would like you to read the rest of the book in your own good time as it will explain how and why the Nysteia Formula works.

At the very end of the book there is an FAQ section.

WE'VE WRITTEN THIS BOOK TO HELP YOU LEAD A HAPPY, HEALTHY, LONGER LIFE; AND WE MAKE YOU TWO PROMISES: FIRSTLY, IT IS THE *ONLY* THING THAT YOU NEED AND SECONDLY IT *WILL* WORK.

CHAPTER 1
HOW YOUR BODY DIGESTS AND USES FOOD

Evolution – Homeostasis – Genetics – Anatomy of the digestive tract – Carbohydrate digestion & metabolism – Protein digestion & metabolism – Fat digestion & metabolism – Energy substrate alternatives – Hormones – Insulin & glucagon – Glycogen – Ketosis & ketone bodies – Krebs cycle – Gluconeogenesis – Autophagy

With most user's manuals it is not really necessary to include information about the inner workings of the product. Similarly, a detailed description of the human body, in particular how it's put together and how it works, is way beyond the scope of this book. For each of these topics, huge text books have been written and it is far more information than you need. We have limited this section to the stuff that is relevant to how the body deals with the food that we put in it.

Evolution

Your body is the most sophisticated creation in the Universe. It is the miraculous result of thousands of biological and chemical processes that have evolved over millions of years.

The theory of evolution, as initially proposed by Darwin, holds that humans have evolved from more primitive life forms. What we have today, in the human body, is a result of a huge number of very small changes to our genes, but large enough to result in a survival advantage. This allowed us to reproduce and pass on these superior genes to the next generation. The evidence in support of this is far more convincing than the idea of creationism which says that the earth and every single living thing on it was created about ten thousand years ago from nothing. The earliest life forms existed on the planet about four billion years ago in fact.

Earliest humans can be traced back to about 150 thousand years ago and over that time evolution has made lots of subtle changes so we now have a much better chance of surviving and living to a ripe old age than primitive man ever did. The consequence is that only the fittest survive. In civilised societies today, we rarely encounter the adverse conditions seen by primitive man. But these survival mechanisms still exist in the human body and are known as homeostatic mechanisms. They are specific biological processes that ensure our bodies function optimally.

Food that is freely available is a very recent thing on this vast time scale. It's only in the last few hundred years that our food has been provided for us by other humans, i.e. farmers. Before this time we had to go out and gather plant food and hunt for animal food every day. That's why we were known as hunter-gatherers.

Today's custom of three meals a day is really very new and is a small blip on that huge time-line. Importantly, the human body and its homeostatic mechanisms did not evolve to handle food in this way. Perversely, the current eating habits of most people in civilised societies should be seen as abnormal and this goes a long way to explaining why the human body has been drawn away from the point where it is functioning optimally to a position where its survival is threatened.

The laying down of fat, both under our skin (subcutaneous) and around our organs (visceral), is a failsafe mechanism that guarantees an alternative supply of energy, in the event that the primary source (glucose) is running low, which happens during enforced fasting or starvation. And this probably occurred often in primitive man whose food supply was far from certain.

The abundant food supply in western societies means this back-up is no longer required because there is always some available. However, the mechanism still exists and explains why the body continues to deposit fat as a storage facility, despite it being surplus to requirement. Importantly it explains why we develop obesity. To counter this, we have to return to how the human body used its energy sources and that means fasting for a large part of the day and this explains how and why intermittent fasting is the most efficient and biologically proven way of getting down to your BOW and staying there.

Homeostasis

Homeostasis is the term given to the large number of systems that exist in the human body to ensure it survives. They operate constantly and, in an adverse environment, aim to bring a particular function back to normality and ensure that the body is performing optimally.

These mechanisms have evolved over a long period of time. Homo sapiens (present day humans) originate from more primitive life forms and our earliest ancestors can be traced back several millions of years. All of the carefully controlled systems within our bodies have evolved over that time, making very small adjustments. What exists today is a reflection of all of those fine tunings.

A good example of a homeostatic mechanism is the way the hormones insulin and glucagon carefully control our blood sugar, making sure that any glucose that is taken in beyond our usual needs is not wasted – it is converted to fatty acids and then stored as adipose tissue (fat). It also ensures that it does not drop below a critical level because certain cells, such as brain cells, must have a ready supply of glucose.

Another important homeostatic mechanism is of course the body's ability to use fatty acids as an alternative source of energy. And intermittent fasting is simply making use of this in the management of obesity. It is, in effect, denying the body its primary energy substrate, and forcing it to use its secondary energy substrate which it gets from stored body fat. It has no alternative and it will happen if you simply allow it to.

Genetics

Your genes are a series of molecules that dictate, amongst other things, how your body is put together and how it works. In each and every cell in your body there are 46 chromosomes that exist as pairs – 23 have come from your mother and 23 from your father. They are assembled from four bases that are in a very specific order and this equates to the various genes. In all there are 3 billion base pairs that make up the genes in each cell.

You can begin to appreciate, therefore, that the control mechanisms are incredibly sophisticated. But importantly we all come from the same gene pool and so there are very, very few differences in our genes which means that your body is almost identical to the complete stranger standing next to you on the bus. And this has important implications in the way your body handles the food you put into it and your response to common illnesses.

Here's a very good example that shows how similar we are to each other: surgeons must know the anatomy of the human body as if it's second nature. And they do this using Gray's Anatomy which is the definitive anatomy text book, (as opposed to Grey's Anatomy the TV program whose name is a parody of the text book, and when it comes to sophistication, bears absolutely no resemblance!). There are close to seven billion people on the planet but, because we all come from the same gene pool, it means that only one version of Gray's Anatomy is needed.

Exactly the same applies to the way our bodies handle food and it is precisely for this reason that we know for sure that if you adopt a certain method of eating then your body will behave in a predictable way. We know that if you fast intermittently and you limit the intake of refined carbohydrate, such as sugar, you will reach your BOF and BOW. If you are above your BOW then you will lose about 1kg a week until you reach it.

When it comes to obesity, as discussed in chapter 3 (body storage of food), your genes are doing exactly what they are supposed to do – to store excess food in the form of fat. There is no doubt that 'genetics' does have a say in whether you have a greater chance of developing obesity but to suggest that it's our genes that have gone wrong is ludicrous. We shouldn't hide from the fact that the vast majority of us handle food in exactly the same way and explains why obesity occurs in so many of us. Obesity is caused by too much insulin, resulting in insulin resistance (IR). Our genes may also make us more susceptible to the development of IR but that's completely different to saying faulty genes cause obesity.

For any doctor, dietician or nutritionist to say that you need to have a tailored solution for your obesity is simply wrong. Not only is it not required for the reasons already stated but it is totally impractical from a manpower and economic point of view. In more than 99% of us the Nysteia Formula, if applied correctly and honestly, will do exactly what you want it to do and that is really all you need to know!

Anatomy of the digestive tract

When food is taken into the mouth it is broken down by the teeth, a process known as mastication. Our teeth have evolved over millions of years to allow us to eat a mixture of different foods, both plant and animal based. In a word we are omnivores. The food is mixed with saliva which lubricates and helps swallowing, otherwise known as deglutition. Saliva also contains an enzyme called amylase which can break down starch into its building blocks, namely glucose. This explains why, if you chew bread for long enough, it will start to taste sweet.

Swallowing involves pushing the food backwards using the tongue into the throat or pharynx which then joins the food pipe or oesophagus. The oesophagus travels down the chest cavity and as soon as it pierces the diaphragm, which is the muscular sheet between the chest and the abdomen, it opens up into the stomach. The stomach is a specific organ within the abdomen.

The food stays in the stomach for a variable amount of time depending on what sort of meal you've just eaten. A churning action resulting from waves of contraction of the stomach wall, otherwise known as peristalsis, once again helps with the breaking up of solid food.

The pylorus is the name given to the outlet of the stomach. At this point it joins the first part of the small intestine. A meal that is particularly fatty can remain in the stomach for a couple of hours and this is done by closing off the pylorus. This delay in gastric emptying explains why a meal, in particular a fatty meal, can delay the onset of the effects of alcohol. Alcohol is only absorbed into the blood stream from the small intestine and if taken on an empty stomach then it tends to travel straight through without staying in the stomach for any length of time, and its effects are felt almost straight away. Taking alcohol with a fatty meal will delay the onset of its effects.

The first part of the small intestine is called the duodenum. Once the food is in the duodenum it mixes with the first set of digestive enzymes from the pancreas which come down a special tube or duct. The pancreatic duct shares the same opening into the duodenum as the common bile duct which is where bile comes in from the liver (Fig 1).

The liver has many important functions. One of them is to make bile which is the green fluid that is essential for digesting fat. The bile is made by the cells of the liver and is collected in a series of tubes within the liver called the bile ducts which then run down into one main tube called the common bile duct. Off the common bile duct is a side branch called the cystic duct and at the end of the cystic duct is the gallbladder (Fig 1). Any bile that is stored within the gallbladder is pushed out on a regular basis by contractions of the gallbladder itself. The gallbladder acts as a storage organ for the bile, although we are not quite sure why this storage facility exists.

Anatomy of the stomach, liver and pancreas

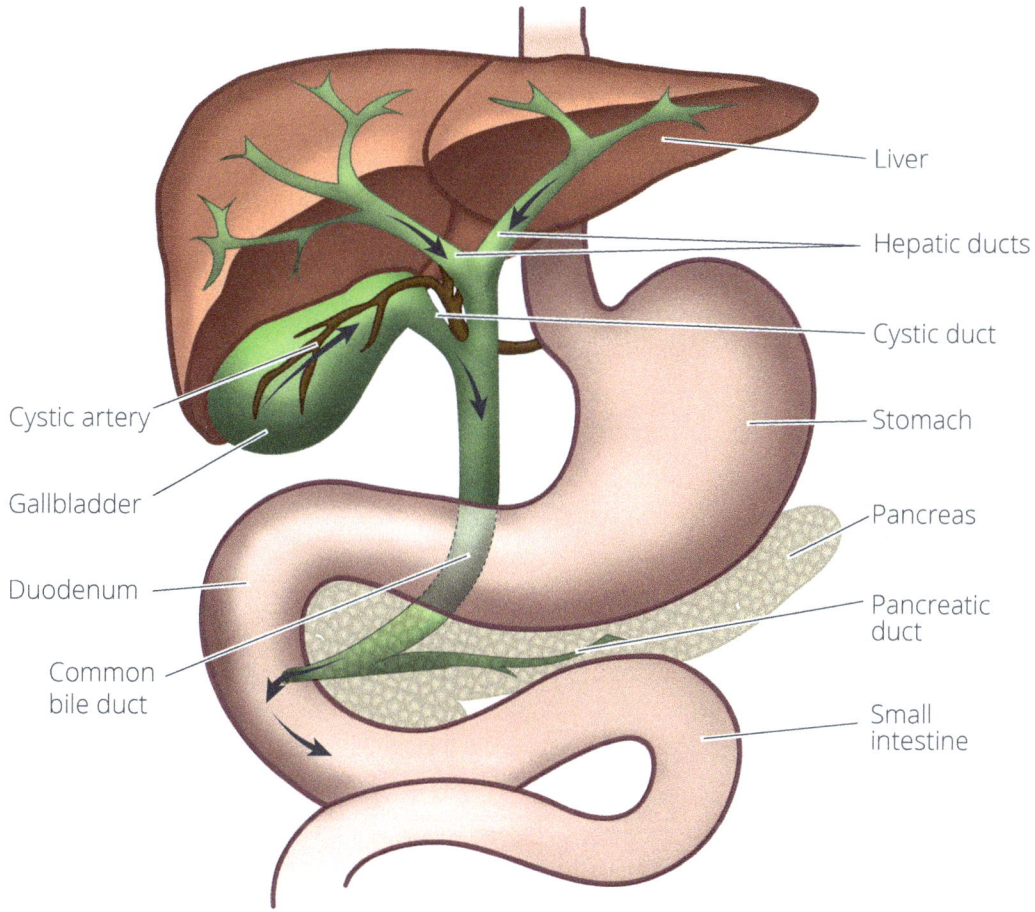

Figure 1. *Anatomy of the stomach, liver and pancreas*

Anatomy of the small and large bowel

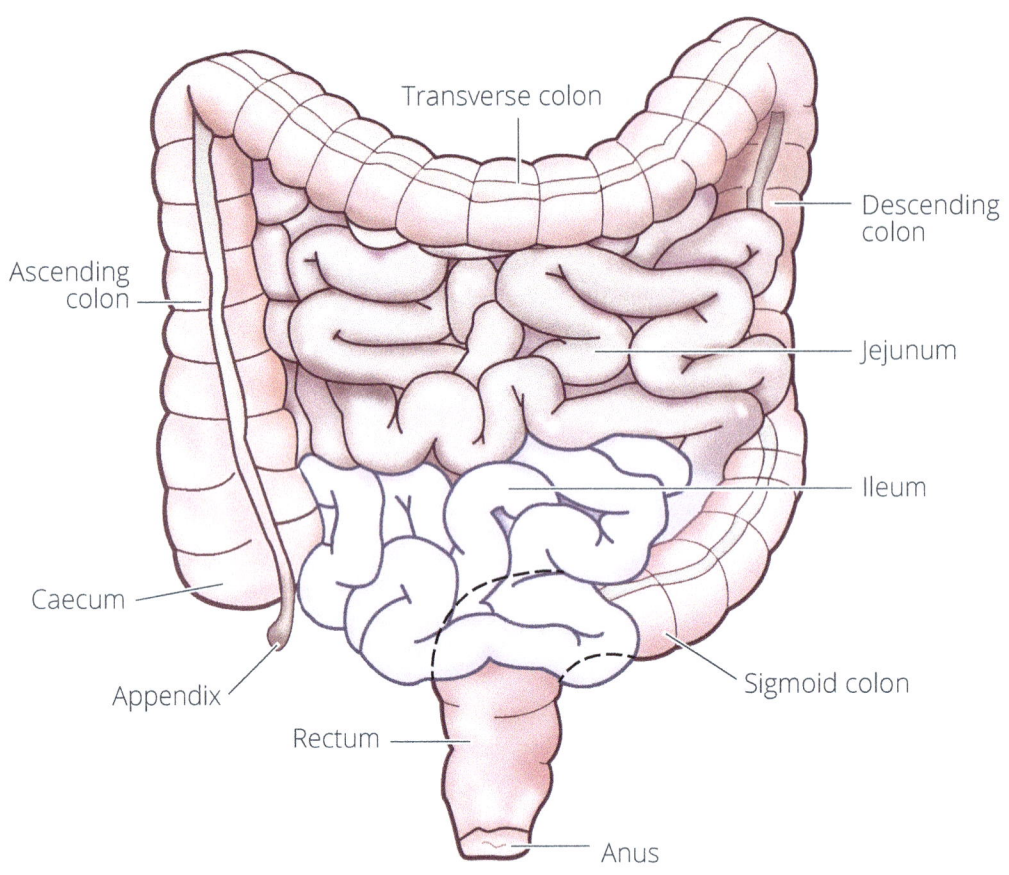

Figure 2. *Anatomy of the small and large bowel*

Once the food has mixed with the digestive enzymes from the pancreas and the bile from the liver it then passes on down through the next part of the small intestine, otherwise known as the jejunum (Fig 2), where enzymatic digestion continues. It then passes on to the last part of the small intestine, known as the ileum.

The products of this breakdown process, namely simple sugars, amino acids and fatty acids, are absorbed through the gut wall into the blood stream to be used by the body. The breakdown of all digestible food should have been completed by the time it reaches the last part of the small intestine, otherwise known as the terminal ileum.

The large intestine is made up of the colon and the rectum collectively. The first part of the colon is called the caecum and is positioned low down in the abdomen on the right-hand side. The appendix, which is an integral part of the gut, is joined to the caecum and this explains why the pain of appendicitis starts here.

The colon consists of numerous parts; firstly the caecum, as discussed, which then becomes the ascending colon (or right colon) which travels up the right side of the abdomen to just below the rib cage close to the liver. It then becomes the transverse colon which travels horizontally across the upper part of the abdomen to a point just below the ribs on the left side and very close to the spleen. It then joins the descending colon or the left colon which travels down the left side of the abdomen. At this point it becomes the sigmoid colon which is so called because it is S shaped. It then passes down into the pelvis where it joins the rectum, which is the last part of the gut.

As previously discussed, by the time the food has reached the terminal ileum, all of the goodness should have been extracted, so all that is left is the non-digestible element of food, in particular fibre. When the waste or faeces is in the caecum it is quite liquid but as it travels around the colon it thickens up because water is extracted from the faeces through the colon wall back into the blood stream. The colon therefore simply acts as a conduit for the faeces which, in the process, thickens up on its way through to the rectum. Colon transit time is the time taken for the faeces to get from the caecum down into the rectum and for most people with a normal functioning gut this is between 12 and 24 hours.

The function of the rectum is to act as a storage organ for the faeces. As faeces are coming through the colon fairly continuously, to save us going to the toilet all the time, the rectum stores up the faeces and typically once a day we get the sensation that the rectum is full at which point we proceed with defaecation. The anus and its associated sphincter complex give us control of the faeces.

Carbohydrate digestion & metabolism

The food we eat is made up of the three macronutrients: carbohydrates, fat and protein. Carbohydrates are divided into two types: complex and simple. Simple carbohydrates consist of single or double sugar units - monosaccharides and disaccharides respectively. Table sugar, otherwise known as sucrose, is a disaccharide made up of a molecule of glucose and a molecule of fructose. Complex carbohydrates contain three or more sugar units linked in a chain. Both simple and complex carbohydrates are digested in the gut by enzymes to glucose.

The glycaemic index, also called GI for short, is a measure of how quickly the blood glucose rises following the ingestion of a certain type of food. Many carbohydrates such as those found in white bread, and some types of white rice and potatoes, have a GI value similar to simple carbohydrates such as sucrose.

Glucose is then transported around the body in the blood stream where it is controlled within very strict limits – somewhere between 4.4 and 6.2 mmol/l. Fasting may drop the lower level marginally and similarly the upper level will rise a little after a meal containing highly refined carbohydrates. It needs to be kept at these levels simply because glucose is the primary energy substrate (energy source) for our cells and therefore a drop to a low level can be dangerous. Conversely a high level will, in the short-term, result in wastage through the kidney. Importantly, in the long-term, raised blood glucose levels, as seen in uncontrolled diabetics, will have a damaging effect on organs such as the kidneys, eyes and blood vessels.

Blood glucose levels are controlled mainly by two hormones that work in harmony but have opposite effects: insulin and glucagon. Secondary hormones also have an effect, including adrenalin, cortisol and growth hormone. Glucose is quickly taken up by the cells to be used for energy, and insulin, a hormone produced by the pancreas in response to a rise in the blood glucose, is essential for pushing glucose into the cells. The role of insulin is covered in greater detail in chapter 4.

Any glucose that cannot be used immediately for energy is not wasted. Instead it is converted into glycogen in the liver and muscles. When this process is saturated it is converted into fatty acids and then stored as body fat. This once again is under the control of insulin. If sufficient glucose cannot be obtained from food that has been ingested, the body firstly calls upon the stored glycogen. This is broken down by a hormone called glucagon. Ingested protein which is broken down into amino acids can be converted to glucose by a process called gluconeogenesis. This once again is promoted by glucagon.

Once the glycogen supply has been used up, and there is insufficient protein to maintain glucose beyond keeping it at baseline levels, via gluconeogenesis, then the body uses its secondary energy substrate. This is fatty acids which, during periods of fasting, are broken down from stored body fat – both subcutaneous and visceral. Understanding this principle is the key to treating obesity and both reaching and staying at your BOW.

Protein digestion and metabolism

Protein digestion starts in the stomach through an enzyme called pepsin and then continues in the duodenum and the jejunum, through enzymes secreted by the pancreas, namely trypsin and chymotrypsin. The proteins are broken down initially into polypeptides and then into their basic units, called amino acids. These are absorbed through the bowel wall into the bloodstream where they are transported into the liver and other cells and used for important cellular functions and to both build and maintain muscle.

The body requires a certain amount of protein for these functions and beyond this it is surplus to requirements. Protein cannot be stored in the body (strictly speaking muscle is not a storage facility in the way that glycogen and fat are) and therefore any excess that is taken in beyond this requirement is broken down in the liver or excreted in the urine. Alternatively, it can be converted to glucose via the gluconeogenic pathway.

Any glucose that cannot be immediately used by the cells for energy or converted to glycogen in the liver is converted to fat and stored as adipose tissue. This explains why a high protein diet runs a significant risk of promoting obesity. The recommended daily intake of protein is about 0.8g per kg of body weight. Therefore, for an average-sized 70kg male this equates to 60g of protein a day.

Proteins are found in both animal and plant foods. The amino acid profile of animal protein is closer to that of humans but all the necessary amino acids can be provided in the amounts required from plant sources. We get most of our protein in the diet from meat, poultry and fish (about 50%), foods made from wheat and similar cereals (25%) and dairy foods (15%).

Fat digestion and metabolism

Fat is an essential macronutrient in that the body requires certain elements that are derived from dietary fats for normal body processes. Secondly, four essential vitamins, namely A, D, E and K, are fat soluble and the absorption of these vitamins is therefore dependent on having some fat in our food.

Most of the fatty acids in the body are obtained from our food in the form of triglycerides that we get from eating both animals and plants. Triglycerides are molecules that contain three fatty acid chains linked to a compound called glycerol. The fatty acids obtained from the fat in land animals tend to be saturated, whilst those in the triglycerides of fish and plants are usually polyunsaturated and therefore present as oil.

Triglycerides cannot be absorbed from the intestine. They are broken down into monoglycerides and diglycerides plus free fatty acids by an enzyme produced by the pancreas called lipase. The fats are then emulsified by the bile salts, produced by the liver allowing the lipase to work optimally at a water-fat interface. They are then absorbed by the cells lining the small intestine where they are resized into triglycerides and then are released into the lymphatic system of the gut. This then drains into the venous circulation and in so doing it does not pass through the liver first, unlike the other products of digestion. Triglycerides, once in the body, are taken up by fat cells (adipocytes), and this is the fat that ultimately leads to obesity, and is what we must force our bodies to use if we want to lose weight.

Glucose that is absorbed from the small intestine travels to the liver via the portal vein. The liver absorbs some of this glucose and replenishes its glycogen stores. It also goes to replenish glycogen stores in the muscles (about 100g and 400g of glycogen respectively, when full). Most of the rest is converted into fatty acids by a process known as lipogenesis which is under the control of insulin. These fatty acids are combined with glycerol once again to form triglycerides in the form of droplets, known as very low-density lipoproteins (VLDL). They are ultimately released, once again, as free fatty acids and glycerol, in the blood when conditions demand, i.e. when blood glucose is at its base line level, and therefore when insulin is low and both glucagon and adrenaline are high.

The cells of the body are required to manufacture and maintain certain cellular structures such as the cell wall and membranes. It is not known wherever they rely for this entirely on free fatty acids that are absorbed from the blood or if they are able to make their own fatty acids from blood glucose. None of the cells in the body can manufacture essential fatty acids which have to be obtained from the diet. Because fat is prevented from entering brain and spinal cord cells (collectively the central nervous system or CNS), these cells have the capability of manufacturing their own fatty acids. Hopefully you can now see why fat in the diet is essential.

Energy substrate alternatives

An energy substrate is any compound derived from our food that is capable of being taken up directly by our cells for the purpose of supplying energy. And that energy is ultimately used for driving the functions of these cells. In effect it is the fuel that the engine runs on. The human body is the most sophisticated being on the planet and has many wonderful mechanisms that have evolved over millions of years. One of these is the ability to use different substrates for cellular energy production. The billions of cells within our body, regardless of their function, use a common pathway for energy production, namely the Krebs cycle (see below).

Because, as previously discussed, the cells of the CNS are unable to use fatty acids, they have an obligatory requirement for glucose as the main substrate. And this of course explains the importance of the biological process known as gluconeogenesis which is the generation of glucose from non-carbohydrate sources (but not fatty acids). It ensures that the supply of glucose never runs out, come what may.

However, the CNS cells are able to switch to using ketone bodies after about three days of starvation. So, in effect this is a failsafe mechanism in the event that the restriction of carbohydrate might extend for longer than usual. Ketone bodies are generated from triglycerides in the liver.

All other cells are able to switch from glucose to fatty acids as an energy substrate with considerable ease. And this of course is the rationale behind intermittent fasting and in particular restricting refined carbohydrate, in the management of obesity. All carbohydrate is converted to glucose in the gut and is absorbed as such. If you don't give the body carbohydrate then effectively you do not give the cells the opportunity to use glucose as its primary substrate.

The cells are also able to use protein as an energy substrate in the form of amino acids, and certain amino acids can enter the Krebs cycle at various points of the cycle. So, there is the opportunity also for dietary protein to be used directly. But, as discussed previously, you have to be aware that a diet that has a lot of protein, runs the risk of switching off lipolysis and thus losing the opportunity of using its stored fat.

Hormones

The hormones found in the body are a group of compounds that act as a control mechanism for the vast number of processes occurring in the human body every second of the day. They are part of the numerous homeostatic mechanisms, all of which are there to ensure these processes function optimally and therefore, from an evolutionary standpoint, we have the best chances of survival. Most of these hormones act via a feedback loop and the best way of illustrating this is to use an example. And what better example than the control of blood glucose.

Insulin is the hormone that is produced by the beta cells in the pancreas and is released from the cells in response to a rise in blood glucose. It is absolutely essential that our blood glucose is maintained within fairly strict limits (4.4 – 6.2 mmol/l). When we eat food containing carbohydrate, it is broken down in the gut and is absorbed into the body as glucose. A rise in blood glucose will promote insulin secretion from the pancreas. The function of insulin is to push the glucose into the individual cells via the insulin receptor for energy. If it cannot be used straight away then it is converted to triglycerides and stored as fat.

When the blood glucose begins to fall the insulin secretion from the pancreas is shut off and glucose levels return to a point within that narrow band. If the blood glucose begins to fall below the lower limit of normal then a second hormone called glucagon, produced by the alpha cells in the pancreas, is released. Its function is to promote a process called gluconeogenesis which is the production of glucose from non-carbohydrate sources, mainly amino acids and glycerol. This is of vital importance because, as previously discussed, the CNS has an obligatory requirement for glucose. It is unable to use the secondary substrate that the rest of the cells in the body are able to use, namely fatty acids.

Other examples of hormones are adrenalin, cortisol, and growth hormone. These are worth mentioning because in fact they are produced in situations when the body needs energy rapidly. In primitive man this was necessary when food was scarce and he needed to go out and hunt and gather for some more. Typically, this was first thing in the morning and this explains why once again from an evolutionary perspective, these hormones are released in greater quantities at this time of day. Importantly they act in exactly the same way when we introduce intermittent fasting as a way of countering IR and obesity. Many people think that if they don't have breakfast first thing in the morning they will simply fall over in a big heap. These hormones act to ensure that quite the opposite happens. In fact, the body is both physically and mentally much more alert in the fasted state, thanks to these hormones.

Insulin and glucagon

Both insulin and glucagon are heavily involved in how the body handles food, especially carbohydrate. Because this aspect is so crucial to the development of obesity, through IR, we have dedicated a separate section (chapter 4) to how these hormones operate and the consequences when it all goes wrong.

Glycogen

Glycogen is a polymer (much like a wall built of identical bricks) of glucose and is a form of storage in both the liver and muscles. When excess carbohydrate is eaten and converted to glucose, beyond what is required for immediate use as energy, instead of being wasted it is converted into glycogen. This process actually occurs in the liver and muscles themselves and is called glycogenesis. You can read about glycogen in more detail in chapter 3 which describes how the body stores food.

Ketosis and ketone bodies

Ketosis is the term given to the body's mechanism of producing ketone bodies. These are three compounds derived from fatty acids – acetoacetate, beta-hydroxybutyrate and their spontaneous breakdown product acetone. Unfortunately, there is considerable confusion amongst people who should know better, namely doctors, dieticians and people in the business of nutrition, as to what ketosis actually is and how it works.

The term is now used to mean diets that are low in carbohydrate, and both for intermittent fasting and starvation. So, we now have a situation where these types of diet are otherwise known as ketogenic diets, suggesting that the production of ketone bodies is the most important factor. Nothing in fact could be further from the truth. Undoubtedly ketosis and the generation of ketone bodies is a normal homeostatic mechanism but it isn't something that needs to happen in order to bring about weight loss.

In addition to glucose and fatty acids, the cells of the body are also able to use ketone bodies for energy, but it is only rarely that these are required. All cells in the body, except the CNS, can switch between glucose and fatty acids. Certainly, in the short term these cells have a requirement for glucose. Gluconeogenesis is the failsafe mechanism that ensures the supply of glucose never runs out and this is through the production of glucose largely from protein. But to avoid the risk of the body using too much of its stored protein in muscle, during periods of short supply, these cells are able to use ketone bodies after about 3 or 4 days of starvation. To lose weight therefore it is not important to induce ketosis, nor is it desirable because it implies that the body is undergoing starvation. This in itself is bad mainly because it reduces the BMR.

The one thing that you really want to happen is to force the body to start lipolysis which is the breakdown of triglycerides in stored adipose tissue into fatty acids and glycerol. Fatty acids can then be transported via the blood stream to all the cells of the body and then to be used effectively as the primary energy substrate. This process can only happen in the absence of insulin. And this explains the rationale for points 1 and 3 of the Nysteia Formula namely intermittent fasting for approximately 18 hours of the day and Mediterranean-type cuisine, together with putting a strict limit on refined carbs. When done every day you will lose 1kg of weight a week.

In reality the three different processes involved in the supply of energy to the cells, namely glycolysis (glucose production), lipolysis (release of fatty acids), and ketosis (production of ketone bodies), is almost certainly happening in parallel (side by side), as opposed to in series (one after the other). The extent to which each of them is happening very much depends upon the supply of carbohydrate and as previously mentioned, for the purpose of weight loss, it is only really necessary to induce significant lipolysis. And this is much easier than trying to induce significant ketosis.

Krebs cycle

The Krebs cycle was identified in 1937 by Hans Krebs and is the key metabolic pathway that connects carbohydrate, fat and protein metabolism in the cell. Knowing how it works is really useful in understanding how the cells of the human body actually use the various energy substrates, and how we have evolved to use an alternative to glucose. It will help in understanding the best and easiest way to tackle obesity.

Krebs cycle

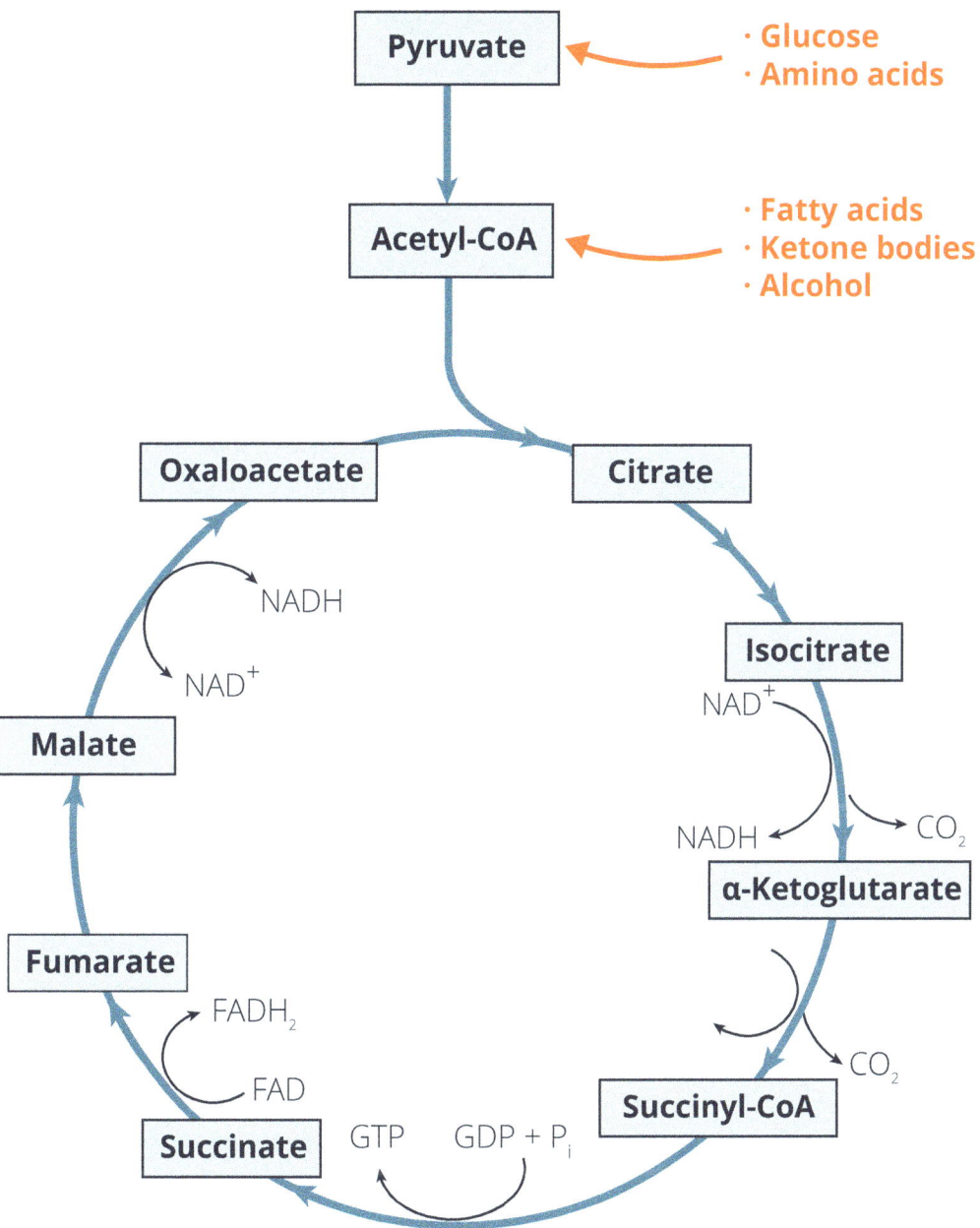

Figure 3. *Krebs cycle*

The molecules in the cycle are converted to other molecules by 8 different enzymes that completely oxidize acetate, in the form of acetyl-CoA, into two molecules each of carbon dioxide and water (Fig 3). The really good thing is that you don't need to know the names nor chemical formulae of these different molecules – merely an understanding will do. In the process, energy is generated which is then used to power the cellular processes that are occurring constantly in our body. Whilst glucose is the primary substrate for the Krebs cycle there are a number of locations where fatty acids and amino acids can enter the cycle, allowing both to be used as body fuel.

In addition to supplying fatty acids, the process of lipolysis (the breakdown of triglycerides in fat) also produces glycerol which itself can enter the cycle. Fructose which is an important component of sucrose or table sugar, can also enter the cycle easily. It is for this reason that the intake of fructose, which is also found in abundance in fruit, needs to be limited so that the body has no alternative but to use fatty acids, resulting in the loss of body fat and therefore weight.

Both ketone bodies and alcohol enter the Krebs cycle by firstly being converted to acetyl-CoA. This explains how drinking a lot of alcohol contributes to obesity. Finally, several amino acids derived from protein can enter the Krebs cycle at various steps, by having the amino group removed. This makes ammonia as a waste molecule which is then converted to urea and this is then excreted in the urine.

Gluconeogenesis

Gluconeogenesis is the body's way of making its own glucose. It does this by using certain non-carbohydrate compounds including glycogenic (glucose producing) amino acids from the breakdown of proteins and from glycerol which is one of the breakdown products of triglycerides. Fatty acids themselves do not enter the gluconeogenic pathway but instead enter the Krebs cycle as an energy substrate in their own right.

Gluconeogenesis exists to maintain blood glucose levels, come what may. Even if we are forced to endure starvation for weeks it ensures an uninterrupted supply. It is promoted by hormones, in particular glucagon and adrenaline. Importantly it prevents hypoglycaemia, or low blood glucose levels, which in reality can only happen with an overdose of insulin, given by injection.

Autophagy

Autophagy literally means the body eating itself. It is the body's way of getting rid of cellular components that are old, damaged, malfunctioning or harmful. In the process they are broken down into basic elements such as amino acids which healthy cells can then use as an energy source. Think of autophagy as the true "detox" the original detox, gifted from evolution, allowing ancestors to survive, even in brutal, primitive times. Remember, we are all descended from people who survived ice ages, when food was scarce (and carbohydrates were almost non-existent). These ancient survivors had bodies that allowed them to store food as fat efficiently – critical in times of food scarcity. Humans who could not easily store fat simply starved to death and were left with no descendants. We now live in a time of great food abundance and, at the same time, we have the genetic predispositions of our ancient ancestors.

When autophagy occurs, the body selectively breaks down unnecessary cellular components, which the body biologically knows it doesn't require for survival. Regular eating reduces autophagy – over many months and years. But with regular fasting, autophagy eats the unnecessary and harmful old stuff and stimulates the growth of new healthy cells. The body thus can become functionally younger – just like new flowers are stimulated to grow, by pulling off the old ones from the plant. Autophagy only happens in a fasted state. The body jealously protects vital organs (e.g. brain, heart and liver) from the initial effects of autophagy, and prioritises the breakdown of superfluous cells and proteins for energy, essentially giving a backup energy source to its own fat reserves in times of fasting by burning the rubbish it doesn't need.

Autophagy might also explain why diseases such as cancer are more common in people who have obesity and why intermittent fasting helps the process. If the body is being denied food for certain parts of the day, as with intermittent fasting, it's easy to see how it could seek out potentially harmful elements to use as a source of energy. In effect it is selectively using its bad cells as food. The opposite is where the body is being over-fed, or has more nutrient than it requires, as in someone with obesity. Now, it has no requirement to use damaged cells for nutrition, allowing them to multiply unrestricted.

This is why many scientific studies have shown that when any living organism is subjected to fasting, it results in a dramatic lifespan increase for that organism – life fights to live in the absence of food. Many scientists believe the only way to naturally lengthen any living thing's life is by stopping it from eating for a period of time.

CHAPTER 2
THE FOOD THAT YOU EAT

Carbohydrate – Protein – Fat – Mediterranean-type cuisine – Micronutrients – Fibre – Alcohol – Measurement of food energy – Daily energy requirements – Intermittent fasting – Weight loss vs weight maintenance

---

Humans have evolved as omnivores which means that we can digest animal and plant products with equal ease. We have the teeth and digestive processes to prove it. A diet that has a good mix of food types provides us with all the essential things we need to keep us healthy. If we choose to eat any other way then we run the risk of deficiencies and illness.

The food we eat is divided into macronutrients and micronutrients. Macronutrients are defined as a class of chemical compounds that we consume in the largest quantities. They provide us with the bulk of the energy that we need to perform all our bodily functions. Micronutrients are essential items in our food such as trace elements and vitamins that make up only a small amount of our intake.

The three main types of macronutrient are carbohydrate, protein and fat. Water makes up a large part of our total diet but it does not provide any nutrition and as such is not classed as a macronutrient.

Carbohydrate

Carbohydrate is found in much of the food we eat. In a typical western diet most of our carbohydrate comes from grain and its refined products such as flour and high fructose corn syrup, and from sugar cane and its refined product in particular sucrose or table sugar. Vegetables, which should make up a large part of everyone's diet, consist mainly of carbohydrate and fibre and in this respect they can be regarded as a "friendly" form of carbohydrate. The glucose-providing part makes up only a proportion of the total, and importantly produces a relatively shallow insulin spike because of the time taken for the gut to digest them. This is the concept of GI or Glycaemic Index which is discussed in the section entitled "carbohydrate digestion". Other sources of carbohydrate include dairy (milk, yoghurt and ice cream), fruit, pasta, bread, rice, legumes (beans), starchy vegetables and sugary sweets, amongst others.

Carbohydrate is broken down in the gut into its constituent molecule, glucose. Each gram of glucose provides the equivalent of 17KJ of energy (1 Calorie = 4.2KJ). And whilst carbohydrate supplies our primary energy substrate, ironically it is the one macronutrient, of the three, that we can dispense with totally. This is because glucose can also be manufactured in the body from protein by a process called gluconeogenesis as described in the previous chapter.

Additionally, and importantly for the purposes of burning fat and losing weight, the body can use its secondary energy substrates in the form of fatty acids and ketone bodies, from both ingested and stored fat. Excess glucose can be converted to triglycerides – and is the process by which we store excess body fat, promoting obesity.

If you make a concerted effort to limit your carbohydrate intake to the ones you would naturally eat in vegetables, fruit, nuts and dairy, your body can function quite happily on 25g to 50g of carbohydrate per day. This is the level that we recommend that people target if weight loss is their goal, or if they are very overweight. Once you have reached your desired weight, you can be more liberal with carbohydrates. For any guide, official or otherwise, to state that there is a minimum requirement for sugar is both patently ludicrous and reckless.

Ironically, the average person's diet contains more carbohydrate than any other macronutrient. We have evolved over millions of years, and only in the last hundred years have carbohydrates been so abundant. Your body is simply not designed to consume the levels that are seen in the typical western diet, and as a consequence it becomes obese, diabetic and subject to all sorts of illnesses.

Carbohydrates cause the greatest spike in insulin, and a constant bombardment of them in our food causes insulin to be present in higher and higher levels in the body. The body then becomes **"insulin resistant"** - the cliff which millions of people have fallen off – leading to the abyss of obesity and the associated diseases of modern living.

Protein

Protein, as with carbohydrate, is found in a wide variety of foods that we eat. We get most of our protein from animals and that means meat and seafood. Other sources of protein include milk, cheese, yoghurt, eggs, beans and nuts. They are broken down in the gut into amino acids. The building blocks of protein are amino acids and once in the body they are reassembled to maintain muscle and to make compounds such as hormones which regulate body functions.

Amino acids are an energy substrate for the cell in their own right but, as previously discussed, usually act in this way by firstly being converted to glucose via gluconeogenesis. Anything that is eaten beyond this basic requirement is either broken down in the liver and excreted or converted to glucose and if this is not used up straight away for energy then it is converted to stored fat. A lot of people are having protein shakes thinking that it's healthy and will help them lose weight but in reality excess protein intake will simply make obesity worse by the process just described. Each gram of protein provides the equivalent of 17KJ of usable energy for the cell.

Fat

Fat, the third macronutrient is once again, found in many foods. It is found in the following: dairy (milk, butter and cheese), red meat and fatty fish, chocolate, whole eggs, nuts, oils (vegetable oil and olive oil) and avocados. The fats that we eat are either saturated, which are solid at room temperature and usually come from meat, or unsaturated, which are liquid at room temperature and are vegetable-based.

Liquid vegetable oils can be made solid by adding hydrogen and they are then known as trans fats. A typical example of this is margarine. About fifty years ago somebody thought this was a good way of substituting it for butter because they thought animal fats were a major risk factor for heart disease. As it turns out this is almost certainly not the case and, perversely, partially hydrogenated trans fatty acids elevate LDL cholesterol and lower HDL cholesterol, causing more harm than good. Trans fats cause about half a million deaths per year and have just been banned in countries like the US.

Fats are broken down in the gut into their building blocks, fatty acids, and then absorbed into the body where they form an important energy substrate and are an important part of basic bodily functions at a cellular level. Alternatively, they are reformed into triglycerides and stored as fat if you eat too much of it. Fat produces quite a lot of energy compared to carbs and protein, with each gram providing about 37KJ.

Mediterranean-type cuisine

The human gut has evolved to digest all three macronutrients with equal ease. It is therefore unnecessary, purely for health reasons, to exclude one or more from the diet on a long-term basis. Equally, it is unnecessary to eat more of one type, say protein, than the others, with the belief that an excess is in some way beneficial. If you do anything other than "everything in moderation" you can potentially run into problems with deficiencies which ultimately can make you sick.

Mediterranean-type cuisine is a concept that we have developed within Nysteia and is really quite specific. We have deliberately not used the term "Mediterranean diet" for good reason. The term "diet" is used loosely and can also mean a set collection of foods but in the context of obesity it usually means some form of food restriction. Secondly, when they hear "Mediterranean diet" most people think of the food that is eaten by Italians which has a reputation for containing quite a lot of carbohydrate in the form of pasta and bread. In fact, anyone who has travelled to Italy will know that they eat quite small portions of carbs relative to other foods such as fresh meat, fish and vegetables. Perversely, the Italian food that you get in restaurants outside Italy contains much larger portions of pasta and bread. The size of the average takeaway pizza is a perfect example.

Including Italy there are 28 countries that have a Mediterranean coastline i.e. a connection with the Mediterranean Sea, and they all have their own cuisines. The thing that connects all of these countries is the abundant use of fresh ingredients and this is something that we think is absolutely vital when it comes to the food we eat. The other main reason for calling it Mediterranean-type cuisine is that it does not exclude other types of cuisine that are just as healthy such as Japanese cuisine and the food you find in the other countries in south east Asia.

Probably the most important aspect of Mediterranean-type cuisine is the exclusion of sugar, anything with added sugar, processed food (which almost certainly contains some added sugar) and refined carbohydrate. Also, anything with the label "low fat" – the fat has been taken out and sugar added to make it taste better because food is quite bland if the fat has been removed. If you eat any of these it will raise your insulin and if this is done often enough and with big enough portions, you will definitely develop significant IR which of course will promote obesity.

Micronutrients

Micronutrients are required in smaller quantities throughout life and consist mainly of the trace elements and vitamins. The most important trace minerals are sodium, potassium, calcium, magnesium, iron and zinc. There are lots of others without which our bodies would not function normally.

The essential vitamins are the vitamin B group and vitamin C both of which are water-soluble. The other essential vitamins, all of which are fat-soluble, are A, D, E and K. Because they are fat soluble this makes fat an extremely important part of the diet. Fat free food tastes very bland and is potentially dangerous because the fat-soluble vitamins would not be absorbed into the body, leading to deficiencies.

Fibre

Fibre is a very important part of our diet, mainly for keeping our bowels regular. There is very good evidence that it has important health benefits such as lowering cholesterol levels and reducing the risk of colon cancer. It is also known as roughage and is the part of food we get from plants that the body cannot digest.

There are two main types. Firstly, soluble fibre which, as the name suggests, dissolves in water and is readily fermented in the colon into gases and physiologically active by-products. Also, it slows down gastric emptying which results in a feeling of satiety which is helpful if you are trying to lose weight because you feel full for longer.

The other type is insoluble fibre which does not dissolve in water and provides bulking. It absorbs water in the process of moving through the gut and, within the colon, it results in easing of defaecation. Fibre can act by changing the nature of the content of the gut and by changing how other nutrients are absorbed.

Plant foods contain both soluble and insoluble types in varying amounts. The health benefits of fibre are largely through the production of healthy compounds during the fermentation of soluble fibre and also through insoluble fibre's ability to increase bulk and to soften faeces, shortening the amount of time it spends in the gut. Because of the gas produced in the colon, as a side effect of the action of bacteria on fibre, it tends to cause bloating which can be a problem if you suffer from irritable bowel syndrome.

Soluble fibre is found in all plant foods, but good sources include legumes such as peas, soy beans and other beans, together with oats, rye, chia and barley. It is also found in fruits including figs, avocados, prunes and ripe bananas. It is found in vegetables such as broccoli and carrots, in psyllium husks and flax seeds. Nuts are also an important source of soluble fibre – almonds contain the highest percentage of soluble fibre of all nuts.

Sources of insoluble fibre include legumes, together with nuts and seeds and wholegrain foods such as wheat and corn. It is also found in vegetables such as green beans and cauliflower and celery.

The recommended daily intake of fibre is about 30g, and in reality you can never have too much. However, it is important to bear in mind that some foods that are high in fibre are also high in carbohydrates so you have to be careful if you're also trying to lose weight. As mentioned numerous times already, limiting carb intake allows the body to use its stored fat as an alternative energy substrate hence promoting weight loss.

Alcohol

Humans have evolved to metabolise alcohol probably because it is a by-product of the fermentation of some forms of fruit in the gut and has therefore come about through necessity. When we drink alcohol, around 5% is lost through urine, sweat or the breath. The other 95% is metabolised by the cells, mainly in the liver.

The alcoholic drinks that we regularly consume contain ethyl alcohol or ethanol for short. You need to avoid at all costs any drink that contains methyl alcohol or methanol (meths) as this is converted to formaldehyde in the body which is poisonous. It is especially damaging to the optic nerve leading to blindness. Hence the term "blind drunk" because back in the day drinking methylated spirits was a cheap way of getting drunk quickly.

Ethanol is broken down in the body by firstly being converted to acetaldehyde. Acetaldehyde is a poison, but it is rapidly converted to acetic acid which in fact is vinegar. This then enters the Krebs cycle (Fig 3) and in this way alcohol is used by the cells as an energy substrate. But because it is denying the cells the opportunity to use glucose and fatty acids as the primary substrates, this is how it contributes to obesity. The enzyme needed for this is called alcohol dehydrogenase which is largely found in the liver and this is the main site of alcohol metabolism.

Alcohol affects some people differently from others. The main difference is between men and women. If a woman and a man of the same weight drink the same amount of alcohol under the exact same circumstances, the woman will on average have a much higher blood alcohol content than the man. This is because females have much less alcohol dehydrogenase in their stomachs than males. If the same man and woman are given an injection of alcohol instead of drinking it they will tend to have the same blood alcohol content and this is because, when the alcohol is injected, it bypasses the alcohol dehydrogenase in the stomach.

If the kidney and liver are exposed to compounds such as acetaldehyde, as in chronic alcoholics, this can lead to severe damage. It will also most certainly explain why there is a link between drinking too much alcohol and certain cancers. Whilst the message is that alcohol can potentially be dangerous, it is like many things in life a question of balancing the benefits and the risks. Most studies that show a link between moderate alcohol consumption and serious disease such as cancer are almost certainly flawed because they rely on individuals reporting accurately their intake. We know that people are notoriously incapable of this simple task – the figure is generally out by about 100%, so it would be safe to double whatever they say.

The benefit of course of alcohol is the effect that it has on the brain and in moderate amounts this produces euphoria and happiness. It also helps us to see our food as a celebration, and something that should be shared with family and friends, as opposed to just another way of relieving our boredom. The secret is to drink in moderation and to be aware at all times that too much can cause harm that is often irreversible. If you believe that you may have become addicted to alcohol then, in reality, the only solution is abstinence.

So can you drink if you are trying to lose weight? As discussed previously, just bear in mind that in supplying your cells with alcohol as an energy substrate, you are denying them the opportunity to use the fatty acids, stored in your fat, as the go-to energy substrate alternative to glucose.

The other important factor to consider is the type of alcoholic drink. All wines except sweet wines which have retained some unfermented sugar, do not contain any carbohydrates because all of the sugar found in the grape juice has been converted by fermentation to alcohol. Therefore it will have very little effect on your insulin levels and will not affect IR that much. Spirits such as vodka, gin and whisky are the same. However, beer has had some carbohydrate added in the form of hops, and this will affect IR and contribute to obesity. It will also take longer to lose weight using the Nysteia Formula.

Measurement of food energy

Food energy, which is the amount of energy provided by one of the three macronutrients, namely carbohydrate, fat and protein, can be measured using either joules or calories.

A joule is the SI unit of work or energy, equal to the work done by a force of one Newton when its point of application moves one metre in the direction of the force. A calorie is specifically a unit of heat energy and is the energy needed to raise the temperature of one gram of water through one degree Celsius. One calorie equals 4.2 joules. Note that calorie spelled with a small c equals 4.2 joules but Calorie spelled with a capital C (a thousand calories) equals 4.2 Kilojoules (KJ).

When it comes to working out how many calories are in a certain amount of food in the laboratory, the food is ignited and the amount of energy released is measured simply by determining the rise in temperature of a set amount of water. This value can then be shown as the energy that is available for use by the body, either in Calories or Kilojoules.

This figure though is somewhat academic because most foods are a mixture of more than one macronutrient. Also, the way the body handles these calories varies with the three macronutrients. In practical terms not all calories are equal. And this is vital to understanding what we must eat in order to help us lose weight.

The widely held belief that a calorie is a calorie is a calorie is simply wrong. And for this reason, amongst others, you shouldn't become obsessed with calorie-counting.

It's important to have a basic idea of how many calories are in your food, but it's totally impractical to weigh every piece and then to refer to a table.

Daily energy requirements

The total amount of energy that our cells require to do their job every day is called total daily energy expenditure (TDEE). Some people call this 'calories-out', whilst the food we eat is 'calories-in'. Ideally the two should match. However, as discussed later, the two are far from independent, meaning 'calories-in' can determine TDEE.

We usually put the TDEE in the average adult as being between 2000 and 2500 Calories and is made up of BMR plus the amount of energy that we use when we exercise. This is an absurdly simplistic approach to the way we manage our weight, and in fact it is our belief that BMR is a lot lower in someone who has significant IR. How this affects the way you lose weight is explained in much more detail in the next chapter, but goes a long way to explaining why the calorie-restricted diet fails every time. As previously mentioned, TDEE is the sum total of the energy used by the billions of cells that make up our body. All of these cells have specialised functions but how hard they are working is infinitely variable, both between individuals and within individuals themselves. Therefore, trying to measure it in a meaningful and reproducible way is impossible.

The majority of TDEE is made up of the BMR – probably as much as 95% – and equates to maintaining the function of the vital organs such as the brain, heart, kidneys, liver and lungs and also body temperature. TDEE can of course be increased for example by doing 30 minutes of cardiovascular exercise, in the form of a 5km run, by about 400–500 Calories.

Another important determinant of BMR is the number of calories that have been eaten (calories-in). Clinical studies have shown that reducing calories-in has a significant effect on the BMR. The brain senses a limited intake and the body automatically responds by reducing BMR. And this is exactly what you would expect from the most sophisticated being on the planet, that has evolved to survive in the face of adversity.

As a result, you feel cold, tired, slow, hungry, irritable and generally miserable. And this contributes significantly to the failure of calorie-restricting diets in the long term. Fundamentally calories-in and calories-out are not independent variables. Quite the opposite – they are very dependent as just highlighted.

Intermittent fasting

Intermittent fasting (IF) is one of the three elements of the Nysteia Formula, and is exactly as the name suggests – it is having nothing to eat for intermittent periods, routinely. It is absolutely not starvation. Starvation is going without any food at all, usually for several days at a time. A lot of people think that IF is severe calorie restriction on certain days of the week – it's not even this (that should be called intermittent severe calorie restriction). Both of these will definitely result in weight loss in the short-term but neither are sustainable for any length of time and will therefore fail in the long-term. There's a significant risk that you will do yourself harm by running into deficiencies of things like vitamins and minerals, and losing muscle bulk. And as with all calorie-restricted diets, your BMR drops down to fairly low levels making you tired, cold and miserable.

To understand the science behind intermittent fasting and why it works for weight loss, it's important to have an understanding of the how the body uses the various macronutrients that are in food, and also the hormones that control what happens to that potential source of energy at a cellular level. This is covered in much more detail in chapter 4.

With the Nysteia Formula the 24-hour day is split into an 18-hour fasting window and a 6-hour feeding window. This has been done for a very good reason – most people will find an 18 hour fast easy to do and it also allows your body a good opportunity for fat-burning. It has to do this if you're not giving it any glucose, and lipolysis can only happen in the absence of insulin. The minute you eat something, insulin goes up and lipolysis switches off. Opportunity lost! The 6-hour feeding window is also enough time for you to eat your 2000 Calories contained in all of that beautiful food. Because IR has been abolished, your BMR sky-rockets well beyond your calorie intake, you go into a calorie deficit and bingo! The weight comes off.

Most individuals will stop eating at about 7pm and then will fast when they're sleeping until they wake up. It is then simply a matter of continuing with the fast for a further 6 – 8 hours. This means going without breakfast and making your lunch the first meal of the day at about 1pm. You will definitely get hungry during this time but this can be kept at bay by regular cups of black coffee, green tea or just tap water. None of these contain any calories and will have no effect on your insulin.

The other really important thing about IF is its regularity. Humans are creatures of habit, and once you are into a routine of the 18-hour fasting window and 6-hour feeding window it becomes much easier to do. And, in fact, after a couple of weeks it becomes so routine that you just treat it as a normal way of life.

Weight loss vs weight maintenance

The goal for everyone should be to achieve their biological optimum weight (BOW). And this is an essential part of Nysteia's philosophy, which is to live a happy, healthy, longer life – by applying the Nysteia Formula. If you are overweight or suffering from obesity, and you do the Nysteia Formula every day, you will lose about 1kg a week, and eventually reach your BOW.

How long this takes of course depends on how overweight you are when you start. It will also depend on how long you've been overweight for. In essence, the longer you have been in this state dictates your level of IR and this is the one thing you need to reverse, and to re-establish your insulin sensitivity (IS). When you first start progress will be relatively slow. But if you stick to the regime closely then your IS returns fairly quickly, glucose is allowed back into the cell, cellular metabolism, BMR and TDEE all increase dramatically, at which point the weight steadily but surely comes off. Sticking to the Nysteia Formula is absolutely fundamental.

Because we know that carbohydrate, in particular refined carbohydrate in the form of sugar, causes IR, it is simply logical to limit its intake if you want to turbo-charge your weight loss. To help you with this we have added the labels 'Weight Loss' and 'Weight Maintenance' to our recipes on the main Nysteia website. This is a good guide as to how much carbohydrate is in a particular meal. Weight loss recipes generally contain less than 50g of carbohydrate per serving, and the weight maintenance recipes contain less than 100g. It's important to bear in mind that with 'good' carbs, such as vegetables, a significant proportion of the weight is taken up by non-digestible fibre. If you want to get into weighing your food then it's probably safe to double these figures to get the actual weight of carbohydrate that is converted to glucose.

Once you have reached your BOW you have two choices. You can either continue with the Nysteia Formula long-term – and we certainly suggest you do this. Or you can relax a little. The danger of course is that you will relax a lot and return to your bad old ways and the weight will go back on. To reiterate Albert Einstein's definition: insanity is doing the same thing over and over again and expecting different results.

It is fine to be a little more relaxed about applying the Nysteia Formula once you have reached your BOW. But just make sure you monitor your weight every now and then so at the very least you'll know if you are going off the rails. One of the ways of relaxing is to shorten your fasting window by an hour or two on some days. The other way is not be so strict about the amount of carbohydrate in your diet, effectively allowing yourself a little more, and this is where the 'Weight Maintenance' label comes in.

CHAPTER 3
HOW YOUR BODY STORES EXCESS FOOD

Storage of carbohydrate – Storage of fat – Obesity – How much body fat do you need for survival?

As discussed in chapter 1 your body has many sophisticated systems that have evolved over a very long time period, and exist to ensure that we function optimally and have the best chance of surviving when faced with adverse conditions. One of them is the ability to store any excess food. This is energy substrate that we take in but cannot use straight away.

There are separate storage facilities for the three macronutrients – carbohydrate, fat and protein. Muscle is the main reserve supply of protein but, strictly speaking, protein doesn't have a depot facility in the same way that carbohydrate and fat do, and that's because amino acids are not a primary energy substrate. They can of course be used in this way, either by feeding into the Krebs cycle directly, or through conversion to glucose via gluconeogenesis, but it only tends to do this as a backup.

Amino acids are not just the building blocks for muscle – they are essential for many critical processes within the cell, hence the importance of eating protein regularly. If the other two depots are getting very low, as in starvation, then it will get it from the breakdown of muscle. This is called proteolysis and results in sarcopenia (muscle wasting) – the unforgettable image of a person living in an area of famine pops up in our brains.

Storage of carbohydrate - glycogen

All the complex carbohydrates in our food are broken down in the gut into glucose which is then is absorbed into the blood stream.

It is then transported to the cells for immediate use. However, if we eat more than we need then it gets converted in the liver and muscles to a polymer called glycogen.
This process is called glycogenesis and is under the control of insulin and other anabolic hormones. Insulin of course is released into the blood from the pancreas in direct response to a rise in blood glucose.

The liver is able to store about 100g of glucose in the form of glycogen, and muscle about 400g – which is equivalent to 2000 Calories worth of energy. This figure is actually very important because if we want to get maximum benefit from our 30 minutes of cardio-vascular exercise (point 2 of the Nysteia Formula) – and that is to deplete our glycogen stores – then it's pretty well impossible to kick-start fat burning if we are constantly topping up our glycogen stores. And this is exactly what's happening with the traditional western diet. If on the other hand you only replenish say a quarter (500 Calories) of the maximum capacity during your 6-hour feeding window then you will deplete your glycogen completely with a combination of an overnight fast and your bout of exercise and then you're straight into using your fat.

This is an absolutely essential step in the management of obesity.

If there is any remaining glycogen in the liver and muscles then the body will use this first. It is broken down by a process called glycogenolysis into individual glucose molecules which will then be used as a primary energy substrate. Lipolysis will not happen until all the glycogen has been largely used up. It certainly won't happen if both blood glucose and glycogen are constantly being replenished, and this of course happens every time you eat another meal containing more carbs. This is also the rationale of point 3 of the Nysteia Formula – Mediterranean-type cuisine – which limits your intake.

Both glycogenesis (the production of glycogen from glucose) and glycogenolysis (the breakdown of glycogen into glucose) are under the direct control of some very important hormones: insulin, glucagon and adrenaline. Insulin's primary role is to control blood glucose and glucose metabolism by pushing glucose from the blood into cells for immediate use. It also promotes glycogenesis.

Glucagon and adrenalin have the opposite effect – they promote glycogenolysis in the liver and muscles into glucose molecules when blood glucose is at its baseline level or during periods when you need energy quickly such as sprinting.

Storage of fat – adipose tissue

The fat in our bodies does two important things: it acts as storage and as protection especially the fat around our organs (visceral fat). But compared to the protection offered by muscle and bone, in reality it provides relatively little protection against anything major like a knife wound for instance. It might act as a cushion but really nothing more than that.

Primitive man's food supply could never have been certain and therefore a storage facility was vital for survival. And this still exists in our bodies today – any fatty acids that are taken in and are surplus to our immediate energy needs are transported to subcutaneous and visceral fat and reassembled as triglycerides and stored there. Additionally, any glucose (and importantly fructose) that is absorbed over and above our ability to store it as glycogen is also converted to fat and stored the same way. This is under the control of various hormones, but insulin is the main player.

How readily this happens varies from person to person and because it's under the control of our genes some people believe that their fat deposition is in some way the result of faulty genes. But this is definitely not the case – certainly not in the vast majority of us. We all come from the same gene pool and there are very few differences in our genetic make-up as discussed in the section about genes in chapter 1. There may be minor variations but, in reality, these genes are doing exactly what they are supposed to do – to store food for a rainy day.

Fat is a very good source of energy backup: each gram releases the equivalent of 9 Calories. So 1kg releases 9000 Calories. If you're using up 2000 Calories a day then that would keep you going for more than four days without the needing to take in anything else. And if you have significant IR and your BMR is down at 1500 Calories, then an extra 10kg of fat will keep you going for two months, without the need for eating anything at all!

Obesity

Obesity is a medical condition where you have so much excess body fat that it may significantly affect your health. Many studies have shown a linear relationship between the level of obesity and both morbidity (illness) and mortality (death), and obesity is one of the leading preventable causes of death worldwide. So, we now talk of someone suffering from obesity, the definition of which is objective, rather than being obese which is both descriptive and subjective.

Two thirds of the adult population in western societies are overweight with half of this group suffering from obesity. Quite apart from the effects on our physical health it takes an enormous toll on our psychological health with a huge number of people simply wishing they could be in the normal range. Thankfully this is easy to do when you've been given the right information.

There are a large number of different medical conditions that are more common if you are suffering from obesity. These include type 2 diabetes, certain cancers in particular the common ones such as breast and bowel, hypertension or high blood pressure, cardiovascular disease such as heart attacks and strokes, and osteoarthritis which is wear and tear on our joints. All of these conditions and others are covered in much more detail in chapter 8.

Body fat can be measured in a number of ways but for the purposes of definition, body mass index (BMI) is used. The most accurate way is when it is measured as a percentage of total body weight (PBF). A healthy adult male has approximately 10-12% PBF and females 11-13%.

BMI is calculated by taking the weight of the person in kilograms and dividing this by the square of the height in metres. So a person who weighs 70 kilograms and is 175cm tall will have a BMI of:

$$70 \div (1.75 \times 1.75) = 23$$

Your BMI is then used to classify your level of obesity in this way:

below 18.5	underweight
18.5 to 25	normal
25 to 29.9	overweight
30 to 34.9	class 1 obesity
35 to 39.9	class 2 or severe obesity
over 40	class 3 or morbid obesity

BMI has largely been developed for social reasons and dividing obesity up into the various categories is artificial because it is in fact a continuous spectrum involving the same process, and that is having too much body fat. The terms "excess lipodeposition" or "adiposity" would be more accurate but, for the sake of consistency, we will stick with the traditional terminology for the time-being.

The use of BMI has its critics but overall, for 95% of us, it is a reasonably accurate and easy way of assessing obesity. The main detractors are people who struggle with the truth and this is based on feelings of guilt which need to be dealt with when managing it. And as with most things in life there's always help from others!

How much body fat do you need for survival?

As previously discussed the body's ability to store excess food is a survival mechanism. But how much fat do you actually need for survival? Well If you are living in a country like the US or Australia where our next meal is no more than two metres away in the fridge or, if you're too lazy to prepare anything yourself, then ten metres away in the form of the front door where the delivery boy will pitch up or, failing that, at the very most fifty metres down the road in the form of a convenience store or fast food outlet, then almost none.

If you are carrying too much fat then we call this being overweight or having obesity and this accounts for at least 65% of us if you use BMI. We say at least because from a survival point of view we believe there is an ideal PBF that equates to our best chance of survival – and this is having just enough in reserve but not so much that it slows us down when we are chasing the woolly mammoth. This is between 10-12% and possibly a percentage point or two higher in women because they have slightly more in the pelvis probably to protect the pelvic organs and the unborn child.

This equates to being at your biological optimum function (BOF) and your biological optimum weight (BOW). And if you want to talk about BMI then it's about 20 which is the lower end of the so-called healthy range. To illustrate the point another way, a 60-year-old male, 175cm tall, living a western lifestyle and having a PBF of 10% will have a BMI of 20 and will weigh 60kg. Importantly he will be at his BOF and BOW, his blood pressure and cholesterol will be normal, he won't be taking a single prescription medicine, and his disease risk will be at a minimum.

A graph of PBF against per head of population will show a standard bell-curve distribution. But he is sitting way down to the left on the x-axis, because only 1% of males his age has less body fat. We would argue therefore that the other 99% have more fat than they need. The irony is that most people would say that he looks far too thin, but that's because our idea of what's healthy has been skewed just like the bell-curve.

But does it actually matter that you have more fat than you need? Well there are two things to consider: how you look and how your body works. Now it doesn't really matter to us how you look but clearly this is a very big source of unhappiness in the vast majority of people who have too much fat. This unhappiness goes as far as anxiety, stress and even clinical depression. And let's not kid ourselves that we don't care about the way we look. The business of dieting is a multi-billion-dollar industry, operated largely by a bunch of snake-oil salesmen preying on your vulnerability, ignorance and insecurity without even hinting at the truth.

Therefore, just our appearance alone affects our health indirectly – big time. But what about how obesity affects our health directly? Well there are now very good statistics that show you are at much greater risk of twelve different types of cancer, heart attacks, strokes, hypertension, arthritis, Alzheimer's, diabetes, OSA and a whole range of inflammatory conditions. The list goes on.

If you are unlucky enough to get struck down with any of these conditions then there's a very good chance you will die prematurely. And in the process you will be a burden to yourself by having to go through some very unpleasant treatments; and to your family and friends, and also to the wider community by using up some very expensive resources.

It all comes down to whether you are prepared to embrace this personal responsibility. If you're not then there's no need to do anything differently. If you don't want to do things differently then you have to accept that you will always be the same and you also have to accept that you stand a very good chance of dying prematurely and miserably and being a burden to everyone around you. Your choice. But if you do want to embrace this responsibility then that means changing, in particular your PBF. And to change that means doing things differently.

The really good news is that to change you really don't need to do things that wildly differently. To achieve and maintain your BOF and BOW, which equates to maximum IS, you only need to do the Nysteia Formula.

CHAPTER 4
INSULIN AND WHY INSULIN RESISTANCE IS SO CRITICAL

Insulin – Control of blood glucose – The role of insulin – The primacy of glucagon – Diabetes – Insulin resistance – Insulin resistance is the gate-keeper – The laws of physics – Why the calorie-restricted diet fails – Elimination of insulin resistance and why the Nysteia Formula works – Insulin resistance is normal – The Renaut Hypothesis

Insulin

Insulin is a naturally occurring hormone, made and secreted by beta cells in the pancreas. Its main function is to deal with glucose once it's in the body having firstly come from the carbohydrate in our food. It was discovered in 1921 by Canadian physician Frederick Banting and medical student Charles Best. They injected the hormone into a dog and found that it lowered high blood glucose levels to normal. Bizarrely, almost a century after the discovery of insulin, doctors continue to overlook the importance of limiting carbohydrate intake when treating diabetes, particularly type 2.

Control of blood glucose

Controlling the amount of glucose in the blood is absolutely vital for survival which, like all the survival mechanisms in the body, has evolved over hundreds of thousands of years. Insulin and glucagon, the other hormone involved, have largely opposite roles and act in harmony.

Normal blood glucose levels sit within a range. When fasting this should be between 4.4 and 6.2 mmol/l. After a meal, especially one that has a lot of carbohydrate, for many people it will rise temporarily to 7.8 mmol/l (hyperglycaemia) but then should drop back to normal levels within a couple of hours. This in fact forms the basis of the standard test for diabetes – the Glucose Tolerance Test. A value between 7.8 and 11 mmol/l indicates "pre-diabetes", whilst a value above 11 mmol/l is diagnostic of diabetes. More information on diabetes can be found both later in this section and in chapter 8.

A blood sugar below 4.4 mmol/l – otherwise known as hypoglycaemia – simply won't happen in the normal person. The light-headedness some people may feel when first applying the Nysteia Formula is not hypoglycaemia; it's just the brain saying "I'm not used to this new routine". And this disappears after a couple of days. The only way a normal person can become hypoglycaemic is if a doctor inadvertently injects them with too much insulin!

The main reason why it is essential to keep blood glucose at this strict level is simple – the brain and spinal cord (collectively the central nervous system or CNS) must have an uninterrupted supply. Unlike the rest of the body, they are unable to use fatty acids which is why we have a very sophisticated mechanism, called gluconeogenesis, that ensures, come what may, the supply of glucose doesn't run out. The CNS can in fact use ketone bodies, through ketosis, as a backup but this only kicks in after about three days of starvation. More information about gluconeogenesis and ketosis can be found in chapter 1.

The role of insulin

When glucose is absorbed through the gut wall into the bloodstream, its baseline level rises. The response of the pancreas to this rise is to produce and secrete more insulin.

Insulin's primary role is to push the increased amounts of glucose into the tissues that need them most – in particular the vital organs and muscles. They act upon the individual cells in these organs, through a receptor on the surface of the cell, that allows entry of glucose through the cell membrane where it can be used for energy by the cell.

The other major role of insulin is to push glucose into the liver and muscles where it promotes the production of glycogen, which is the storage facility for glucose – a process called glycogenesis. And when the glycogen stores reach capacity, any glucose that is still coming in is converted to triglycerides and stored as fat – a process called lipogenesis – once again under the control of insulin. So you can see that the human body is very efficient when it comes to not wasting any energy substrate, and you can see what an important role insulin has.

How quickly and how high the insulin rises following a meal very much depends on what's in the meal you've just eaten. By far the greatest rise is seen with carbohydrate which is converted to glucose in the gut. A significant but smaller rise in insulin is seen with protein and this happens via a secondary route – any protein that is ingested beyond what is required for normal body functions, such as building and repairing our muscles and producing important hormones, is converted to glucose via a process called gluconeogenesis. This then produces a rise in blood insulin. By contrast fat produces an almost negligible rise in blood insulin. It is essential to appreciate these differences when it comes to understanding what causes chronically elevated insulin levels and how this leads to IR and how this results in obesity; and importantly how to treat it.

The primacy of glucagon

Glucagon is a hormone, secreted by the alpha cells of the pancreas, in response to a fall in both insulin and blood glucose. As previously mentioned, its actions are opposite to those of insulin in that it helps to keep blood glucose levels up by promoting both gluconeogenesis and through glycogenolysis which is the breakdown of glycogen into glucose molecules. Because it is absolutely vital to maintain blood glucose above a minimum level, for reasons already stated, it can be argued that glucagon is the most important chemical in the body – and certainly when it comes to the different hormones in the body. Without it the supply of glucose would stop about an hour after our last meal and we would die very quickly because of the brain's immediate need.

Diabetes

A more detailed description of diabetes can be found in chapter 8. It is discussed briefly here because its development – both type 1 and type 2 – is very closely related to insulin.

Type 1 diabetes is an autoimmune disease where the cells in the pancreas that produce insulin are destroyed by the body's own immune system. We really don't understand why this happens. The result is that not enough insulin is produced to properly regulate blood sugar – which becomes a lot higher (hyperglycaemia). This glucose then gets lost in the urine and is therefore wasted.

Patients with type 1 diabetes tend to be very skinny as they can't store fat efficiently (insulin promotes lipogenesis). They also suffer from the long-term effects of chronic hyperglycaemia and that is cardiovascular disease, renal failure and eye disease leading to blindness. The treatment of type 1 diabetes is to control blood glucose levels by injecting insulin. It has to be given by injection because it is a protein and would be broken down in the gut, just like any other protein, if given by mouth.

Type 2 diabetes shares the same problem as type 1 diabetes i.e. uncontrolled blood sugar levels. However, in contrast, the levels of insulin in the blood are greater than normal. So, in fact the body is producing too much insulin. It does this in response to IR which itself develops as a result of significantly elevated levels of insulin secondary to the almost constant supply of carbohydrate from the diet. This then sets up a vicious circle, where the body's response to IR is to produce even more insulin. And so the process continues.

In type 2 diabetes, because there is IR, insulin is in fact unable to do its job – the cells of the body become resistant to it. They don't respond the way they should. This allows blood sugar levels to rise above the normal range and the individual then suffers exactly the same consequences as patients who have uncontrolled type 1 diabetes, namely heart disease, kidney failure and eye disease.

The traditional treatment of type 2 diabetes is to help the body to produce more insulin in the form of medication, initially using pills. And when this fails, insulin needs to be given by injection. Perversely, this does exactly the opposite to what we want to see which is to get rid of IR. It simply amplifies the vicious circle and makes things worse.

It is vital to appreciate that the only way to break the vicious circle of insulin further promoting IR is to let the body do what it has evolved to do. That is to reduce insulin secretion by the pancreas and the only way this can be done is by dramatically cutting back on carbs, either on its own or ideally combined with intermittent fasting.

Insulin resistance

Insulin resistance (IR) is exactly what the name suggests – the cells of the body become resistant to its actions and do not respond to insulin as they would do when the body is in a state of optimal function. As mentioned earlier, insulin is produced by the pancreas every time we have something to eat. The size of the response very much depends on what's in the food and we refer to the glycaemic index (GI) which is a way of measuring this. High GI foods produce a much greater insulin response than low GI foods. And this is very much related to the actual amount of glucose that's released from carbohydrate after it's broken down in the gut.

Primitive man never really ate high GI foods, as the majority of such foods have been developed by agricultural practice quite recently. Let's now fast forward several hundreds of thousands of years where modern man has plenty of food generally, and too much high GI food specifically. In western societies the supply is never in doubt. But the body processes that have evolved over this time still exist. Now, every time blood insulin is elevated, which of course happens especially with high GI foods such as sugar and refined carbohydrate, this promotes IR. If you eat a similar meal soon after, more insulin is needed to do the same job, and that's to keep blood glucose inside the strict levels of 4.4 to 6.2 mmol/l. But at some point, when the pancreas is pushing out as much insulin as it can, this won't be enough, and glucose levels exceed the upper limit and this of course results in diabetes. This is shown schematically in the following set of images (fig 4).

The blue line is increasing carbohydrate intake, and the red arrows show the insulin response which then moves the cells along the IS/IR cursor. IR then determines how much glucose goes into the cells for immediate energy use and how much gets converted to triglycerides and stored as body fat, and this is shown in Fig 5.

Carbohydrate consumption determines insulin response and insulin resistance

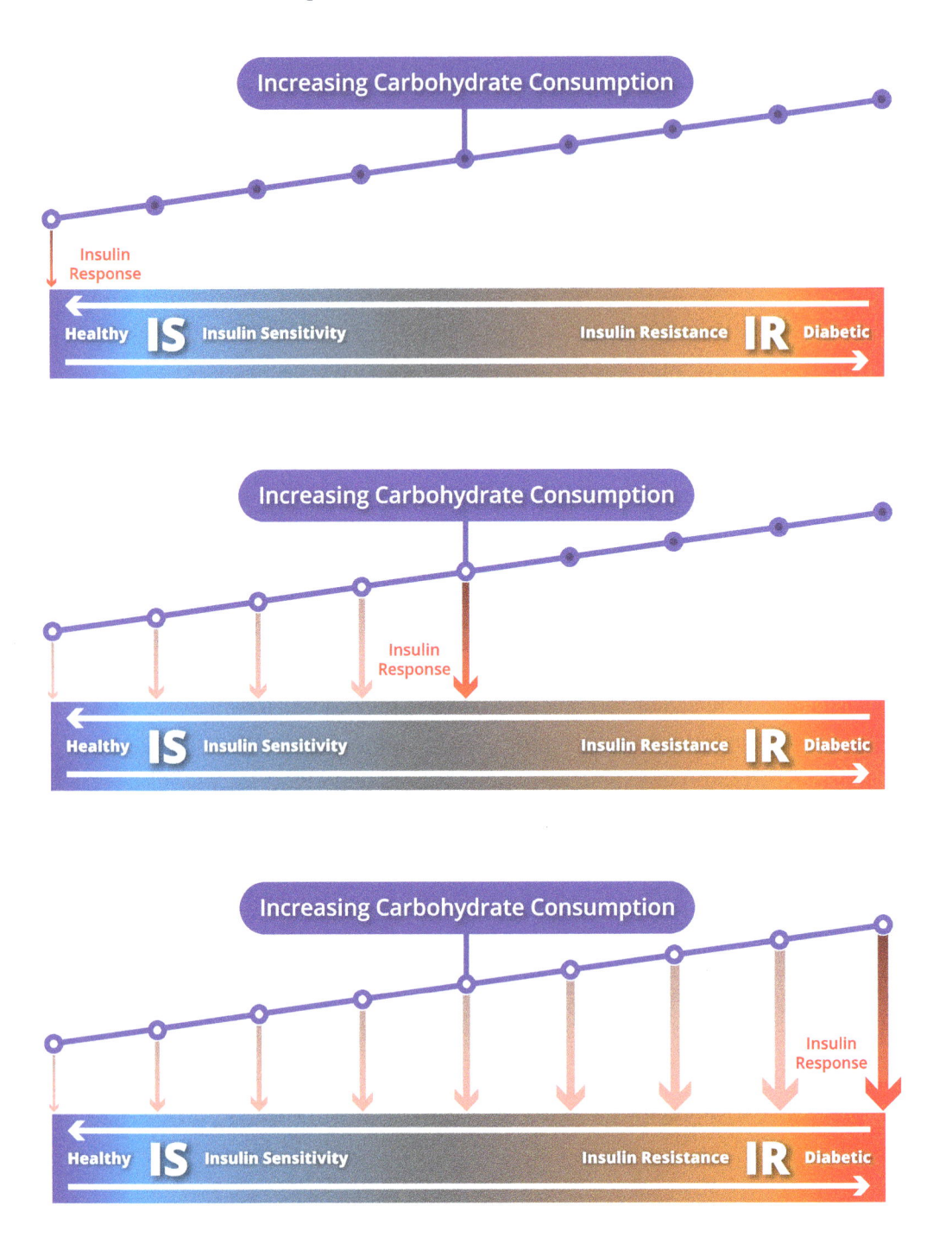

Figure 4. *Carbohydrate consumption determines insulin response and insulin resistance*

Insulin resistance determines where glucose goes – into cells or fat storage

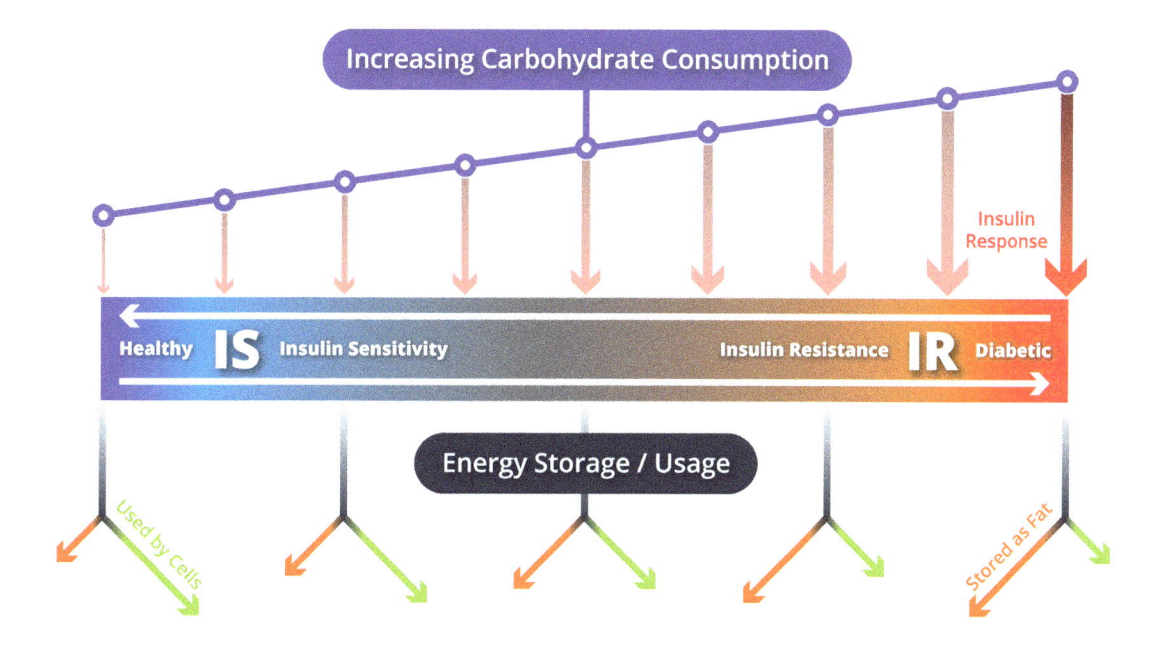

Figure 5. *Insulin resistance determines where glucose goes – into cells or fat storage*

Insulin resistance is the gate-keeper

Figures 6 and 7 show the fate of carbohydrate once it has been broken down and absorbed as glucose into the blood stream, and how IR determines in which direction it goes. It has three possible pathways: directly into the billions of different cells in the body for immediate use, polymerisation to glycogen for storage in the liver and muscles (glycogenesis) or conversion to triglycerides which are then stored as fat.

If you have eaten lots of refined carbohydrate over many months and years you will have significant IR and you belong in Fig 6. Glucose can get into your cells but it's finding it relatively difficult because IR has partially closed the gate. The insulin receptor is responsible for allowing glucose through and, at a molecular level, it's probably down-regulation of the receptor itself, through IR, that facilitates this. As a consequence, the glucose that is available is limited and the chemical reactions within the Krebs cycle slow down and, with it, energy production. Which means the cell is no longer functioning optimally, and the overall effect is to drop your BMR.

Because the body doesn't want to waste the glucose that you've just eaten, it shunts it in the direction of its storage facility. It does this by converting it to glycogen which is then stored in the liver and muscles. As previously discussed, this storage facility is really quite limited – when at capacity there's about 100g and 400g respectively which can supply the equivalent of approximately 2000 Calories. Once it is at capacity, and if you continue to eat even more carbohydrate, then it has no alternative but to send it in the direction of lipogenesis which is the conversion to fatty acids which are then stored as triglycerides in your subcutaneous and visceral fat.

You're probably thinking at this point that if glucose can't get into the cell because of IR then it can always use the stored fatty acids. Here's the really bad news: it can't because this requires lipolysis to happen and any amount of insulin will switch off this process. The cell is effectively starved of all its substrate and the overall effect is to put the body into a mini-hibernation.

If you continue to eat this way then you're merely perpetuating the process – IR is maintained by the pancreas being forced to secrete a constant supply of insulin, glucose is unable to get into the cell, glycogen stores are constantly being topped up, and the majority gets stored as fat which the body is not able to access.

In contrast, if you have no IR, and therefore maximal IS, Fig 7 is the most likely scenario. The insulin receptor is up-regulated and the gate opens. The glucose you've just absorbed has no difficulty getting into your cells, allowing it to enter the Krebs cycle, resulting in maximal energy production, optimal cellular function and a high BMR. If any glucose or fatty acids that you've just eaten are completely used up then, as always, you can call upon your glycogen stores and fat stores. Glycogenolysis and lipolysis proceed unhindered because your insulin levels are at zero.

Importantly, your brain and body are fully connected and talking to each other about how much food you need to eat to maintain the necessary supply of energy substrate, be that glucose or fatty acids. The vast majority of what you eat will go straight into your cells for immediate use. Only a small amount will go in the direction of glycogenesis and in reality you only need about a quarter of this quick-access facility. Almost none, if any, will go in the direction of lipogenesis, so you'll never put on weight.

The idea that insulin resistance is the gate-keeper is exactly that – and it forms the basis of the Renaut Hypothesis, as described shortly. Anyone is allowed to trash our hypothesis and we invite individuals, scientific groups, research laboratories and universities who have pots of money, and the facilities, to do just that. But in the process they are required to submit an alternative hypothesis that would adequately explain what we are seeing in practice. Continuing with what we currently believe and what we are practicing is not an acceptable alternative, because that's clearly not working – the problem is getting bigger by the day. Literally.

The idea is based on pure logic; and here's the really good thing – in practice it works, just by applying the Nysteia Formula. Intermittent fasting eliminates insulin resistance by keeping insulin at zero for most of the day, aided by Mediterranean-type cuisine which restricts the intake of refined carbohydrate. Only a small proportion of your glycogen storage facility is being utilised and any that is being replenished is being used up with the combination of an overnight fast and a thirty-minute bout of cardiovascular exercise first thing in the morning. If you then continue the fast for a further six hours then your cells have no alternative but to use your stored fat as an energy substrate, which they can of course now do as zero insulin permits lipolysis. Could it be any simpler?

Energy storage / usage of carbs in a person with insulin resistance (IR)

```
Carbohydrate consumption
          ↓
   Absorbed as glucose
```

promoted by insulin

- lipogenesis → **glucose coverted to fat** — adipose tissue
- glycogenesis → **glucose converted to glycogen** — liver & muscles
- blocked by IR → **glucose used by cell** — low BMR, FA used by cell

blocked by IR — glycogenolysis

lipolysis (blocked by insulin)

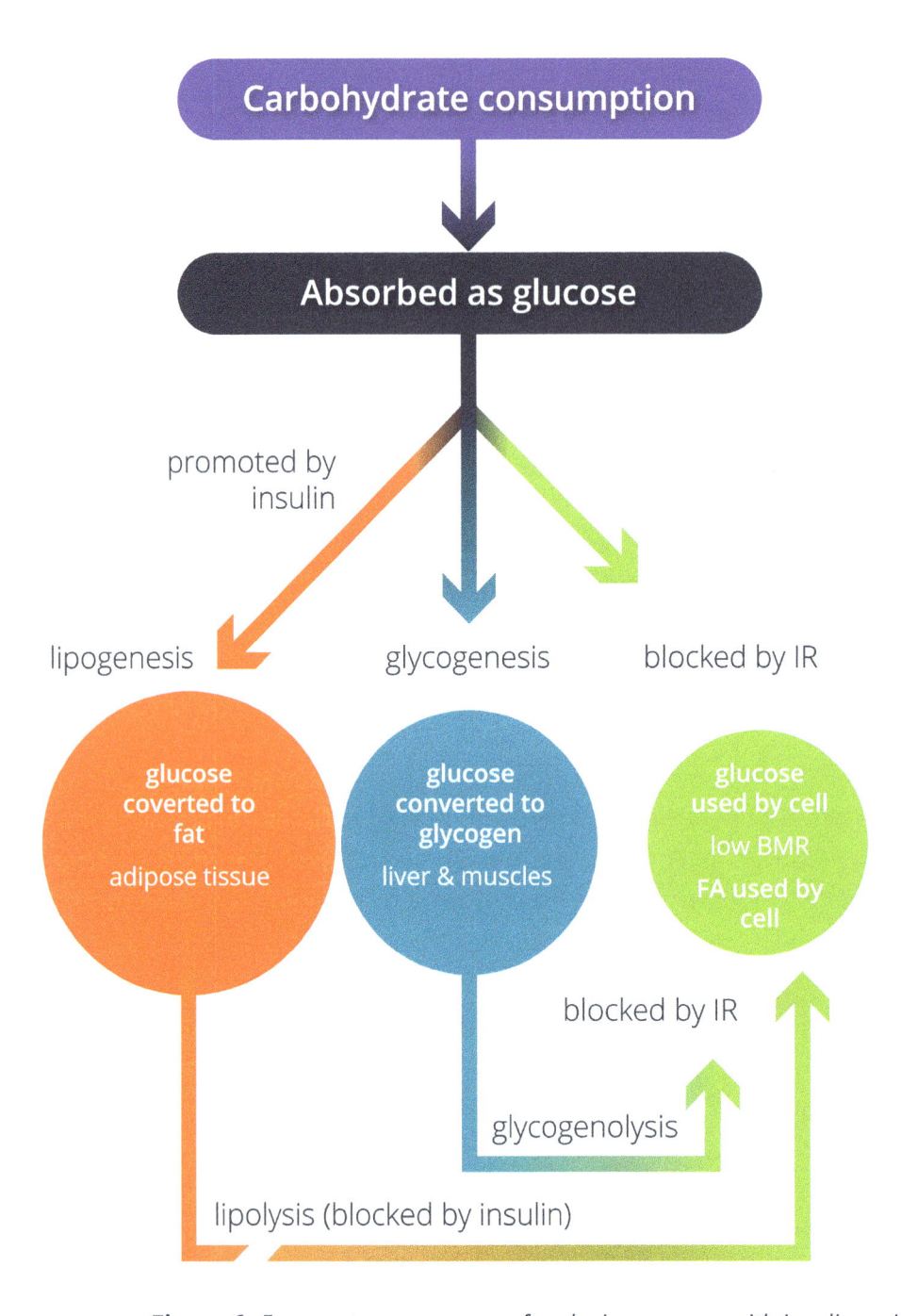

Figure 6. *Energy storage - usage of carbs in a person with insulin resistance*

Energy storage / usage of carbs in a person with insulin sensitivity (IS)

Carbohydrate consumption

↓

Absorbed as glucose

promoted by insulin

- lipogenesis → **glucose coverted to fat** — adipose tissue
- glycogenesis → **glucose converted to glycogen** — liver & muscles
- → **glucose used by cell** — high BMR, FA used by cell

glycogenolysis

lipolysis (blocked by insulin)

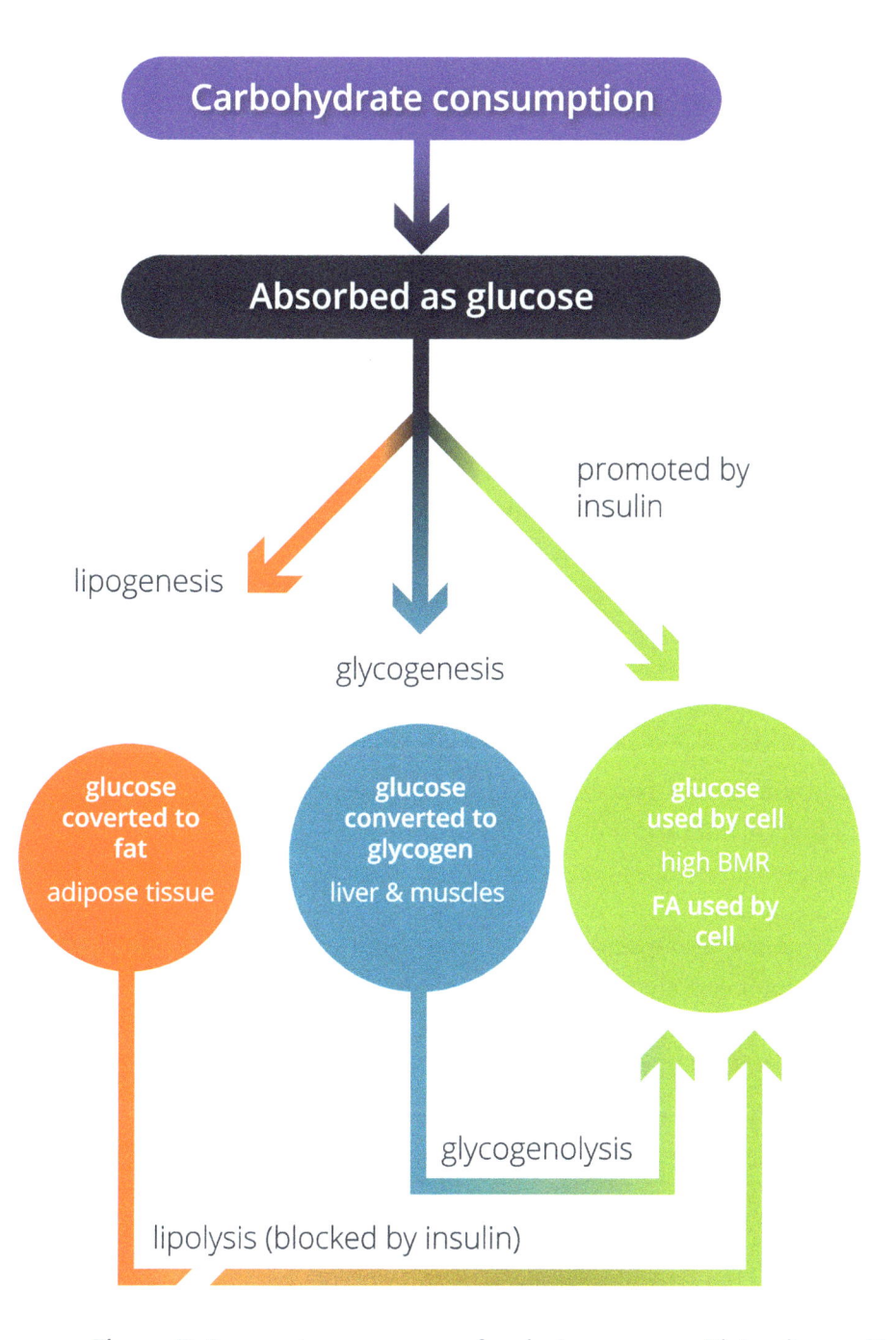

Figure 7. *Energy storage - usage of carbs in a person with insulin sensitivity*

The laws of physics

The first law of thermodynamics states that the total amount of energy in the universe is constant – it can neither be created nor destroyed – it can only be converted from one form to another. And this applies to the human body because effectively it is an isolated entity, For it to stay in the steady state, energy used (calories-out) has to equal energy supplied (calories-in).

As described previously, if you eat more food than you need for immediate use, the potential energy in that substrate isn't wasted or dispersed. It is instead converted to a form that the body can store. If we then want to force our bodies to use the energy that is held in that storage facility we obviously need to limit further intake. But we also need to make sure that calories-out are greater than calories-in. There is certainly no problem in measuring intake (although it becomes quite tedious to do it for every meal), but when it comes to expenditure we come across two major problems – firstly it's impossible to measure accurately and even guessing can by wildly out. Second, the brain has the ability to sense that intake has been cut and responds by shutting down body processes that are not critical for survival. This is exactly what you would expect from the most sophisticated being in the Universe, in particular one that has evolved over a long period of time to survive.

If your body uses its stored fat as an energy substrate then, yes, you will lose fat and lose weight – the goal of any diet. But if you are still limiting or severely restricting your intake and you're not losing the weight as expected, that can only mean one thing – your expenditure, i.e. BMR and therefore TDEE, are very low. We call this a "slow metabolism". And the thing that determines this is your level of IR.

Fig 8 shows how fat deposition starts and how it continues. The typical person at the top end of the healthy BMI range will start eating too much. This happens for a number of reasons including boredom, unhappiness, peer pressure and the ready supply of fast food. That in itself will cause you to put on weight but the thing that turbo-charges it is the drop in BMR as a result of IR. You will have a moderate amount of IR already but it is dramatically increased by the pancreas being forced to push out ever-increasing quantities of insulin. This is the inevitable outcome of eating big portions of refined carbs, at regular intervals.

How fat deposition starts and continues

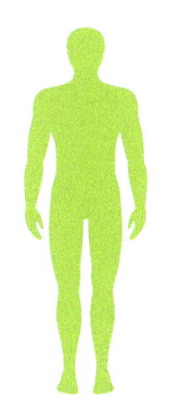

Start phase

2500 Calories

BMR: 1700
Exercise: 100
TDEE: 1800

- large, frequent meals with large quantities of refined carbs
- limited exercise
- moderate IR with low BMR
- brain and body disconnected, no communication re: intake
- energy surplus of 700 Cal / day
- weight gain of 80 g / day

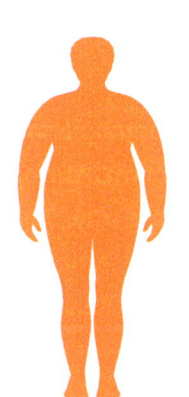

Intermediate phase

2500 Calories

BMR: 1500
Exercise: 100
TDEE: 1600

- large, frequent meals with large quantities of refined carbs
- limited exercise
- increasing IR with very low BMR
- brain and body disconnected, no communication re: intake
- energy surplus of 900 Cal / day
- weight gain of 100 g / day

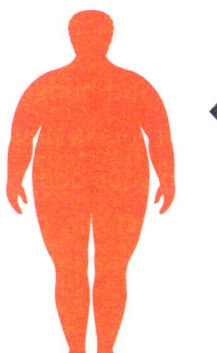

Continuation phase

2500 Calories

BMR: 1500
Exercise: 0
TDEE: 1500

* All figures listed refer to Calories.

- large, frequent meals with large quantities of refined carbs
- no exercise
- significant IR with very low BMR
- brain and body disconnected, no communication re: intake
- energy surplus of 1000 Cal / day
- weight gain of 110 g / day

Figure 8. *How fat deposition starts and is continued*

Because the weight has gone on and because IR is restricting the supply of glucose to muscle cells, any exercise that you did before is now far too difficult, so you simply stop, dropping TDEE even further. Even if you make a conscious effort to reduce intake, because the equation is still stacked very much in favour of energy surplus, the weight continues to be piled on. To reverse this, you firstly have to get rid of IR; and this explains beautifully why the calorie-restricted diet fails and why using the Nysteia Formula (NF) is the only realistic and sustainable solution.

Why the calorie-restricted diet fails

The traditional "weight loss diet" is the calorie-restricted diet which is numerous small meals, generally high in carbohydrate, taken at frequent intervals. Bizarrely, so-called experts are undeterred by the clinical evidence that clearly shows it doesn't work in the long-term; and anyone who has tried a calorie-restricted diet will know from bitter experience this is the case. That goes for any method of weight loss that doesn't specifically address IR. Fig 9 shows how and why this happens.

If you are overweight or have obesity you will have a low BMR (a "slow metabolism"). You wrongly assume that your TDEE is about 2000 Calories. There's no way of measuring it in a meaningful way, but let's say you are actually using 1500 Calories a day. The traditional calorie-restricted diet will typically put you on an intake of say 1200 Calories, and because the first law of thermodynamics applies, there's an initial weight loss of a few kilograms. But your brain then senses that intake is being restricted and will shut down your body even further to match the intake, giving you an even lower BMR. Hence the plateau that everyone experiences. And you will remain at this plateau for as long as IR is being maintained which of course it now is – by the frequent small meals you've been told to eat.

You're now thoroughly miserable because you are cold, exhausted, slow and hungry. So what do you do? – you start eating again of course. And because your intake now exceeds expenditure the weight goes back on and, because of the lag in your body's ability to reset its BMR back to where it was before the diet started, you actually put on more weight than before. This is the yo-yo effect that anyone who has been on a calorie-restricted diet experiences.

Why weight loss fails with the calorie restricted diet

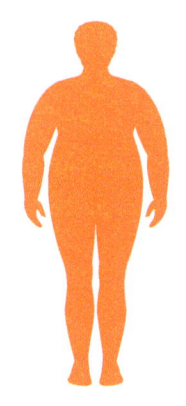

Weight loss phase

← 1200 Calories

BMR: 1500
Exercise: 100
TDEE: 1600

- small, frequent meals with moderate quantities of refined carbs
- limited exercise
- IR remains high, BMR unchanged
- brain and body partially connected, re: intake
- energy deficit of 400 Cal / day
- weight loss of 45 g / day

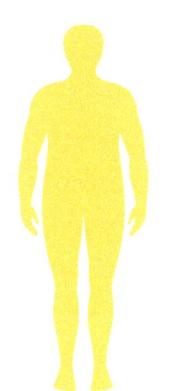

Weight plateau phase

← 1200 Calories

BMR: 1200
Exercise: 0
TDEE: 1200

- small, frequent meals with moderate quantities of refined carbs
- no exercise
- IR unchanged
- brain senses limited intake, body shuts down BMR
- energy expenditure = energy intake
- no weight loss

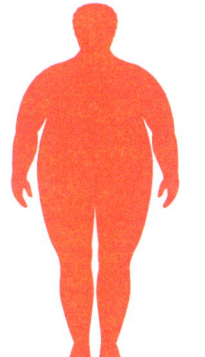

Weight regain phase

← 2500 Calories

BMR: 1200
Exercise: 0
TDEE: 1200

All figures listed refer to Calories.

- large, frequent meals with large quantities of refined carbs
- no exercise
- IR increases to diabetic levels, BMR remains very low
- brain and body disconnected, no communication re: intake
- energy surplus of 1300 Cal / day
- weight gain of 145 g / day

Figure 9. *Why weight loss fails with the calorie restricted diet*

Elimination of IR and why the Nysteia Formula works

If IR is the underlying problem in obesity then clearly the logical answer to losing weight is to get rid of it – that means keeping insulin levels at zero for most of the day. And this is exactly what happens in practice. How do you limit insulin production? – stop eating, in particular refined carbs! The really good thing is that this doesn't mean you need to starve. For reasons already discussed, it's extremely important you maintain intake at about 2000 Calories. The brain tells the body that the intake is good, and this maintains a normal BMR.

This is the rationale for points 1 and 3 of the Nysteia Formula, i.e. intermittent fasting and Mediterranean-type cuisine. For 18 hours of the day, ideally, you're not eating any food, in particular no refined carbs, and the pancreas is not releasing any insulin. This allows the cells to regain their IS. It also gives you sufficient time in the other 6 hours, to eat all that beautiful, fresh, healthy food that you've prepared yourself. And this maintains your BMR.

Figure 10 shows how this happens in practice. A fat person with IR will have a low BMR and low TDEE. By contrast, a fat person without IR will have maximal cellular metabolism but, because of the extra work that they have to do to simply move the body around, together with the necessary biochemical processes, both BMR and TDEE are increased dramatically. Energy expenditure is now much greater than intake, automatically putting the body into a deficit. It might seem counter-intuitive but it's important to keep up intake so that whole-body metabolism is kept at this new elevated level.

Intermittent fasting of course also allows the body to use its alternative energy substrate. And it will get this from stored fat which means most people will lose 1kg per week on average. Lipolysis, which is the body's normal mechanism for releasing fatty acids from stored adipose tissue, can only happen in the absence of insulin. As soon as you eat anything there's an insulin response which will switch off lipolysis straight away. And with it the opportunity for fat-burning and weight loss!

Why weight loss succeeds with the Nysteia Formula

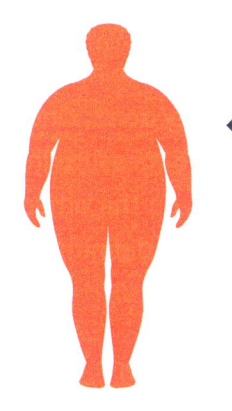

Start phase

2000 Calories

BMR: 2000
Exercise: 700
TDEE: 2700

- intermittent fasting
- Mediterranean-type cuisine
- 30 mins daily cardio exercise
- IR decreasing, BMR increasing
- brain and body reconnecting and communicating re: intake
- energy deficit of 700 Cal / day
- weight loss of 80 g / day

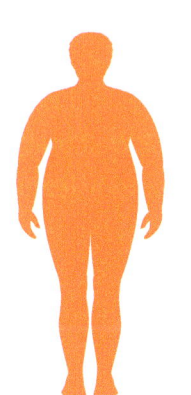

Continuation phase

2000 Calories

BMR: 2300
Exercise: 700
TDEE: 3000

- intermittent fasting
- Mediterranean-type cuisine
- 30 mins daily cardio exercise
- IR rapidly diminishing, BMR boosted
- brain and body reconnected and communicating re: intake
- energy deficit of 1000 Cal / day
- weight loss of 110 g / day

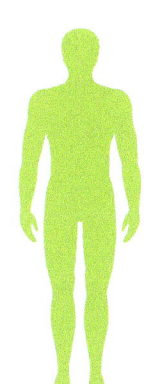

Equilibrium phase

2500 Calories

BMR: 2000
Exercise: 500
TDEE: 2500

* All figures listed refer to Calories.

- intermittent fasting
- Mediterranean-type cuisine
- 30 mins daily cardio exercise
- IR zero, IS maximal, BMR stable
- brain and body fully connected and communicating re: intake
- energy expenditure = energy intake
- BOF and BOW achieved and maintained

Figure 10. *Why weight loss succeeds with the Nysteia Formula*

IR is normal

The vast majority of doctors, nurses and nutritionists looking after people with obesity and diabetes believe that IR is itself a disease and is caused by obesity, either by association or as a direct cause and effect. This has never been proven, which is significant, but a very good reason for dismissing the idea completely is that, if indeed obesity caused IR then everyone who had IR would have obesity. But they don't. One of the problems we have in trying to work this out is that IR is difficult to measure in individual patients (it can only be measured indirectly). Type 2 diabetes on the other hand is quite easy to diagnose and we know that IR exists in all diabetics (by definition). But not all diabetics are obese.

We believe that in fact it's the other way around – IR causes obesity. And the one thing that is very much on our side is that if you get rid of IR, by getting rid of excess insulin, obesity disappears!

We also believe that IR is a normal mechanism that exists to restrict the entry of glucose into the cell. If it's normal that means it must have evolved to help us survive; and now you're asking the really big question: how could it possibly help us survive? Well that's easy – when primitive man had plenty of food he needed a method of both storing it and conserving it. You've just learned in the last chapter how he stored it; the development of IR allowed him to conserve it. A chronically elevated insulin, as seen in the fed state, leads to IR which then does both of these things – it promotes storage and helps to conserve it by putting the cell's "brake" on.

When the food ran out the opposite happened: insulin levels dropped to zero, IR was abolished, full IS was regained, glucose was allowed back into the cells, lipolysis provided a steady supply of fatty acids, BMR sky-rocketed and off he went looking for his next meal. It is yet another example of a superbly orchestrated homeostatic mechanism that has evolved to ensure the survival of the species and it forms the basis of the Renaut Hypothesis.

The Renaut Hypothesis

A hypothesis is another name for an idea. The Renaut Hypothesis states that IR is a normal homeostatic mechanism that has evolved over hundreds of thousands of years as a survival mechanism. It acts to conserve energy substrate by slowing entry of glucose into the cell and to store the excess by converting it to triglycerides and depositing it as fat. Both processes conveniently are under the control of the same hormone – insulin.

Whilst IR may have evolved as a survival mechanism, it certainly wasn't intended to be carried to the point where it is unable to cope with the extremes of modern lifestyles (too much availability and consumption of high GI food) and where it will potentially have an adverse effect on the body. This excessive lifestyle is exactly what we are seeing now in western societies and the body's response to this provides the basis for the Renaut Paradigm as described in chapter 9.

CHAPTER 5
THE REAL MEANING OF METABOLISM, HEALTH AND FITNESS

Metabolism – Control of cellular metabolism – Health and fitness

We often use the terms "health" and "fitness" without really knowing what they actually mean. We also talk about someone being "healthy" and "fit". The problem is they are descriptive terms – there is no good objective way of measuring them with a blood test or diagnostic scan for example.

There are certainly things like blood pressure, heart rate, an ECG, and blood tests that we can do to measure cholesterol, kidney function and liver function. But the reality is that the organs just mentioned, and the body as a whole, have enormous reserve so in fact you can be really quite sick and still have normal results, effectively hiding the true picture. And this explains why people we see as being very healthy can suddenly be struck down with a serious illness and even die prematurely.

Equally we use the term "metabolism" without really giving much thought as to its true meaning. We talk glibly about someone having a "fast" or "slow" metabolism and how some things can "boost" your metabolism. Health, fitness and metabolism, as we shall see, are all closely linked and we can't talk about health and fitness without firstly discussing the finer points of metabolism.

Metabolism

Metabolism is used in different ways and means a number of things. As an example, people talk about it in relation to how the gut handles food – but strictly speaking this is digestion and absorption. Others talk about it in relation to how basic substrates such as glucose are controlled in the blood stream and how they are stored and taken up by the tissues – but this should be called homeostasis.

From a biochemical point of view "metabolism" is really about what happens to a compound like glucose once it's inside the cell and in particular how it feeds into the Krebs cycle for generating the energy that is used for driving the cell's processes.

The body is made up of billions of cells, all having a specialist function; so when we talk about the body's metabolism we are referring to the sum total of the individual cells' metabolism. And because the body is doing different things at different times of the day, the demand on the various cell types is constantly changing. Depending on what you require your body to do, your metabolism is in a constant state of flux.

Truly measuring a cell's metabolism directly, i.e. how much energy it is using, is impossible. We can only measure the body's metabolism, and this is done by measuring the amount of carbon dioxide produced by the lungs because this is the common end product of metabolism at a cellular level. But this is an indirect measurement (essentially a proxy for the actual value) and is undertaken in a very artificial environment because we need to be hooked up to some complicated equipment either in the laboratory or carried on our backs if we are moving around.

There are thousands of biological processes and chemical reactions occurring constantly in our bodies, totally independent of whether we are running around or sitting in a chair, almost all of which are happening automatically without us having to think about them. As an example, our thought processes are a function of our brain cells, and how much energy they are using depends on what we are thinking about – and we are always thinking about something; digestion is a function of the cells that line our gut – and how hard they are working depends on what we've just eaten.

The point is this: our metabolism varies enormously from person to person and within individuals themselves depending on what we are doing. To try and come up with a number is an educated guess at best. As with all educated guesses they can be very wide of the mark and therein lies the problem with calorie-restricted diets.

Control of cellular metabolism

The big question we need to answer is: what controls a cell's metabolism? The chemical reactions and biological processes taking place in a cell are immensely complex; and the mechanisms that control these processes are similarly complex, as you would expect, and well beyond the scope of this book. But a basic understanding is always good.

One of the very basic ways of controlling a cell's metabolism is to limit how much energy substrate it can use and in particular how fast it can enter the cell. As discussed in the chapter on insulin and IR, the insulin receptor allows glucose to get into the cell from the blood stream. How much IR the cell has dictates this. It is there to conserve energy by effectively putting our cells and our body into a mini-hibernation. So, the cells slow down: our muscles cells are slow leading to physical fatigue and our brain cells are slow leading to mental fatigue. All the things that you experience on a daily basis if you are overweight or have obesity. But of course, it's not the obesity that causes this – it's the IR that goes with it.

That said, you can of course have IR without obesity, but this is very much the exception rather than the rule. The important thing to bear in mind is that if you are eating the typical western diet you will have some degree of IR, irrespective of how much body fat you have. And the more IR you have, the more difficult it is to shift the fat. It also explains why the calorie-restricted diet fails every time as discussed in the previous chapter – and that goes for any method of weight loss that doesn't specifically deal with IR. The solution of course is to boost your cells' metabolism and that means getting rid of IR as discussed previously.

Health and fitness

Now that we have an understanding of how IR controls a cell's metabolism we can begin to appreciate how, if this is taken off track far enough, it can result in poor health and a lack of fitness. True health equals mental and physical fitness and these are ultimately down to the function and health of the individual cells. The state of the body is therefore the sum total of these cells' capabilities.

All of these cellular processes rely on a ready supply of energy substrate in the form of glucose or fatty acids. It is our hypothesis that IR is in fact a normal homeostatic process that has evolved to limit the supply of glucose to the cells, effectively putting them into a mini-hibernation when in the fed state to conserve energy. But obviously not enough to adversely affect their function.

If, however you extend IR far beyond its intended limits then you will potentially affect cellular function in a bad way. As an example, it would explain why the cell might no longer metabolise cholesterol properly, leading to high blood cholesterol. Our blood pressure is controlled by specialised cells called baroreceptor cells in the carotid artery – if these don't work properly we get hypertension (high blood pressure). And it would explain the so-called metabolic syndrome which we see in obesity. It isn't the obesity – it's the underlying IR.

Importantly, it supports the Renaut Hypothesis. This, in turn, is behind the Renaut Paradigm which is hypometabolic immune cells secondary to IR leading to disease initiation and repair failure; and would explain why we are more prone to illness – or are less healthy – if we're not eating correctly.

So the relative terms "health" and "fitness" equate to the sum total of cellular health. Biological optimum function or BOF means optimal cellular health and is determined by how readily glucose can get into the cells which in turn is affected by how much IR the cells have. And the latter is determined by how much insulin your body is producing. When you are producing just the right amount you are stabilised at your biological optimum weight or BOW which equates to about 10% body fat. You will remain stable because a state of equilibrium is reached by the body telling the brain how much food it needs.

When you are in equilibrium you are at your BOW, you have maximal IS, you have BOF, you have a PBF of 10%, your disease risk is minimal, your chances of survival are greatest, you are "healthy", you are "fit" and you simply feel fantastic. And the best bit is, to achieve all of this, you only have to apply the Nysteia Formula.

CHAPTER 6
WHY PHYSICAL ACTIVITY & EXERCISE ARE ESSENTIAL

Cardiovascular exercise – Why cardiovascular exercise is so important – Exercise whilst in the fasted state – You will not exercise the weight off – Muscle strengthening

As discussed in other sections of the book, what we have in the human body is a result of evolution – the enormous number of fine-tunings in our genes that have translated into a survival advantage.

Our bones, muscles, joints and ligaments are very much part of that evolutionary process and are there to make us mobile. But if you do things drastically differently to the way primitive man lived and you don't use them then, once again, you're in danger of dismissing that survival advantage. And that's exactly what see with today's sedentary life-style.

Cars, trains, buses, escalators, elevators and moving walkways are now part of everyday life which means we no longer use our skeletal system, except to move around the house and get into the car. For many people that's the sum total. As a result, our muscles lose their tone and become weak and flaccid, our bones lose their strength and become more likely to break, and our joints become less flexible resulting in stiffness and pain. It's called disuse atrophy. It's not just our bones and muscles that suffer either; the systems that support them – our energy supply, our cardiovascular system and even our brain all become less efficient as a consequence.

The irony once again is that it doesn't take a great deal of effort to keep things in good working order. After all primitive man didn't have a treadmill or dumb-bells to help him keep in shape; but undoubtedly he did a bit of walking most days and he used his upper body to defend himself and to build.

Point 2 of the Nysteia Formula is cardiovascular exercise for 30 minutes every day – there's very good evidence that shows this is all you need to do to keep your muscles and bones in optimum health, and also to help you maintain your BOF and BOW and ultimately to live to a ripe old age.

Cardiovascular exercise

Cardiovascular exercise is so called because of the effect that it has on your cardiovascular system which is your heart and blood vessels. It is defined as any physical activity that raises your heart rate.

Normal resting heart rate or HR has a range and this is between 45 and 90 beats per minute. A value outside of this range, when at rest, is abnormal. If it is below the lower limit of normal this is called bradycardia, and if it is above the upper limit of normal this is a tachycardia. There are many conditions that can cause these abnormal values but the usual problem is the heart's very own nerve supply.

A tachycardia when you're exercising, as opposed to a tachycardia at rest, is quite normal and exists to pump more blood around the body to deliver more oxygen and nutrients to the cells that need it most i.e. the muscles. How much blood the heart pumps out is called the cardiac output or CO and is measured in litres per minute. Each beat of the heart pushes out a certain volume and this is called the stroke volume or SV. With an adult at rest this is usually about 80mls of blood per beat.

Cardiac output is calculated by multiplying stroke volume by heart rate:

CO (litres/min) = SV (mls) x HR (beats per min)

So, you can see that a person with a heart rate of 60 will have a cardiac output of almost 5 litres. If you want to increase the output you can do it by increasing both heart rate and stroke volume and in reality both happen together and this can result in a doubling or even tripling of the cardiac output during strenuous exercise.

Why cardiovascular exercise is so important

When you exercise, the heart pumps out more blood automatically – you don't have to think about it. This is thanks to the sympathetic nervous system and is otherwise known as the "fight and flight" response. It is a normal homeostatic mechanism that has evolved to make sure your body responds when you are faced with potential danger such as a predator. This probably happened on a daily basis in primitive man but thankfully is much rarer now.

However, it's important that you still use this facility regularly so as to maintain that survival advantage and this is exactly the reason for doing cardiovascular exercise. Regular exercise has been shown to have a very positive effect on general health and lifespan. And, of course, the opposite is true as you would expect.

The other very good reason why cardiovascular exercise helps to extend life is that the heart itself consists mainly of muscle: and just like any other muscle if you don't give it a regular workout it becomes weak, flaccid and inefficient.

If you are overweight or already suffering from obesity then it's only natural that you will find any form of exercise difficult, even walking. This is for two reasons: firstly, you are having to carry around an extra 20-30kg every minute of the day, and secondly the IR that has been built up over the years limits how much glucose can get into your muscle cells. But the good news is that even starting with a brisk walk will put up your heart rate. As time goes on your cells will regain their IS and you will steadily lose weight. Your exercise limit increases, so you can walk faster and faster. You will then break into a jog and finally a run.

The answer is to start gently and to build up over time. The important thing is to push yourself a little bit further each and every day so that after half an hour you can feel your pulse racing, you are sweating and you are out of breath – that's how you know you've done some good! If walking and running aren't for you it's important that you find something that is, such as cycling, swimming or going to the gym.

Exercise whilst in the fasted state

You should do your cardiovascular exercise while you're still fasting – don't worry, your body has plenty of reserves and that's exactly what you want it to use. Your immediate energy reserves will be your liver and muscle glycogen stores. If you're trying to lose weight then it's important to get rid of these early in the day and this will happen with a good bout of exercise. You're then into uninterrupted fat burning for a good six hours before you start eating again. The amount of energy your body requires at rest is about 70 Calories per hour. Thirty minutes of cardio activity will cause you to expend about 220 Calories, or 3 equivalent hours of resting energy. When you do your cardio activity in a fasted state, it has the effect of "fast forwarding" your fasting time, in addition to depleting any residual glycogen stores.

If you fast for 18 hours and do 30 minutes of cardio activity as well, your body has used 21 hours' worth of resting energy. It gives more chance for autophagy to increase every day, with its associated many benefits. Cardio activity in a fasted state gives rise to vital opportunities for the body to cleanse and condition itself and reduce insulin resistance over the long term. And it's important that you do it every day for at least thirty minutes – no more excuses!

You will not exercise the weight off

You've probably been told many times that you have to exercise to get the weight off, but in fact exercise by itself will not result in fat loss. It will certainly accelerate the weight loss because it increases your TDEE; but the majority of TDEE is made up of your BMR which is low anyway because of IR. The simple reason why it isn't a long-term weight-loss solution is because, of course, it doesn't fully deal with IR which is the underlying problem in obesity. This can only be done by getting rid of insulin for a significant part of the day and this can really only be achieved by adopting the other two points of the Nysteia Formula, i.e. intermittent fasting and Mediterranean-type cuisine. All three have to be done together in order to achieve and maintain your BOF and BOW.

Muscle strengthening

Most forms of physical activity involve the leg muscles and in the process their strength is maintained automatically. But the muscles of the upper body tend to get neglected so it's important to do some form of simple exercise to help them keep not only their strength but also their tone and definition. It stops things looking flabby. Doing ten minutes of upper body exercises such as push-ups, sit-ups, pull-ups and using some basic equipment like dumb-bells, three times a week, will suffice. Ideally it should be done just after your bout of cardiovascular exercise.

CHAPTER 7
HOW YOUR BODY FIGHTS DISEASE AND ILLNESS

Inflammation & the inflammatory reaction – The immune response – Healing or death – Immune cell function – The Renaut Equation

The immune system is a very sophisticated system in the human body that has evolved, just like all the other systems in your body, over hundreds of thousands of years and plays an important part in your ability to survive in the face of adversity. In this particular case we are talking about injury or more accurately an "insult". We use inverted commas because the term covers just about everything that is potentially harmful. It includes not just physical injury from trauma say, but also an infection caused by bacteria or a virus, or even when we get cancer.

The immune system is designed to deal with all of these insults, so as to get rid of it as quickly as possible, and repair any damage, with the aim of returning the body to optimal function, or as close to normal as possible.

The system is made up of immune cells and a large number of different chemicals that act together. The cells, otherwise known as white blood cells (WBC) or leucocytes, start off life and grow in the bone marrow and other collections of lymphoid tissue (a site where the cells live). The ones we are most familiar with are lymph nodes or glands. But there are lots of others such as in the bowel wall – these are strategically placed to deal with a potential pathogen, such as bacteria that have found their way into our food.

The leucocytes are free to roam in the blood stream with the other main type of cell – erythrocytes or red blood cells (RBC). They are also found in the fluid that bathes our cells, known as extra-cellular fluid, and they can find their way into tissue that has become diseased or damaged such as tumours. Importantly they are attracted, by a clever type of homing mechanism, to a particular site allowing them to interact at close quarters with whatever is causing the problem, be that a virus or cancer cell. The enemy typically displays a protein, called an antigen, that is recognised as foreign. And so begins the complex series of processes and chemical reactions that should eliminate whatever is displaying the antigen. The chemicals that help these processes are called cytokines, or lymphokines when specifically related to lymphocytes.

Inflammation and the inflammatory reaction

Inflammation is the term given to the reaction we see when the body meets something potentially harmful such as an infection. Typically there are some macroscopic changes i.e. things that can be seen with the naked eye, and some microscopic changes that can only be seen with a microscope.

The obvious things that can be seen, and felt, were originally given Latin names by the ancient physicians: tumor, dolor, calor and rubor which respectively are swelling, pain, heat and redness. Together they make up the "inflammatory reaction" and happen because of chemicals released by our own cells in the process of interacting with whatever insult the body is trying to eliminate.

The inflammatory reaction is part of our evolution and exists to increase our chances of survival. It's there to remind us that, whatever has caused it, be it a wasp sting, a cut or an infection, we should do our very best to stay clear of it in the future – the next encounter might be our last!

Ironically, in some cases the inflammatory reaction itself can result in long-term damage. Since the inflammatory reaction is part and parcel of the immune response, it is easy to see how a lengthy and severe insult might have an adverse effect on the body. And as shown below there are two major things that determine the immune response and hence both the inflammatory reaction and the outcome – the size of the insult and how well the immune system is working.

There is now good evidence that, with many conditions, it's not just the insult that's to blame for the damage – part of it is due to an exaggerated inflammatory reaction. A good example is blaming animal fat for the high rate of heart attacks and strokes. Doctors now believe that a key factor is the inflammation in the blood vessel wall leading to an atheromatous plaque which then causes a blockage. The risk is obviously higher if that inflammatory reaction is greater. The atheromatous plaque might have a high fat content, but a high blood cholesterol, which is largely unrelated to fat in the diet, is probably not the culprit.

The immune response

This is the broad term that covers the immensely complex series of biological processes and chemical reactions that swing into action the very second the body encounters an insult, such as trauma, infection or cancer. As previously discussed it involves WBCs and cytokines. We'll talk about the cells because we think IR dictates how efficiently they work which ultimately determines your risk of disease and the outcome.

WBCs include:

T lymphocytes – this subset of lymphocytes is concerned with cell-mediated immunity i.e. there is a one-on-one interaction with foreign cells such as bacteria. The group is further divided into T-helper cells (identified by the CD4 marker) which help other lymphocytes, and cytotoxic T-cells (CD8 marker) that directly kill cells infected by viruses and tumour cells.

B Lymphocytes – this subset of lymphocytes is concerned with the humoral, i.e. blood-borne, part of the immune system. They interact with specific antigens (foreign proteins expressed by viruses, bacteria and tumour cells) and, in response, produce specific proteins themselves called antibodies, or immunoglobulins, that neutralise the potentially harmful agent.

Natural Killer cells (NK) – NK cells are a further subset of lymphocytes that are cytotoxic (cell-killing) but are, however, unique in their ability to recognize stressed cells in the absence of antibodies, resulting in a much faster immune response.

Macrophages – these WBCs engulf and digest cell debris, foreign substances, microbes (e.g. bacteria), cancer cells, and anything else that doesn't have the type of proteins we see in a healthy cell on its surface, by a process called phagocytosis.

Neutrophils – these cells are phagocytes, like macrophages, and are recruited to the site of injury within minutes following trauma and are the hallmark of acute inflammation.

Tumour Infiltrating Lymphocytes (TIL) – these are lymphocytes found within cancers. If a solid tumour, such as a breast or bowel cancer, is taken out, cut up in the lab and then stained for specific markers such as CD4 and CD8, and then examined down a microscope, a whole bunch of cells light up. This proves that the tumour cells express antigens (bad proteins) and that the tumour has been infiltrated with immune cells that are clearly there in an antigenic role i.e. to try and destroy the cancer cells. TILs are almost always present in any solid tumour and whether they are effective in seeing the cancer cells as foreign and destroying them is very much down to how efficiently they are working.

Healing or death

We come from the same gene pool and, as a result, the way our cells function is almost identical. You would therefore expect our immune systems to respond in pretty much the same way when we are exposed to an infection that affects a whole community say. And in reality this is exactly what happens.

How promptly and how effectively your body responds to a potential threat such as a viral infection is very much related to an interplay of the size of the threat, i.e. how dangerous the virus is, and the efficiency of your immune system.

So, that relationship can be written like this:

Disease + Immune Response = Outcome

The term "Disease" covers everything that can affect the human body, including infections, trauma and cancer. "Immune Response" is the efficacy of our immune system, and "Outcome" is whether we recover partially (and are left with a defect or disability) or completely (otherwise known as resolution), or whether we go downhill and die.

Some people fare better than others, when faced with an identical illness. Which means that, whilst the response of the immune system is fairly standard, effective function varies from person to person. We see this even when we think someone is healthy and we expect them to not even suffer from the condition in the first place; if they do, they will recover very quickly. But this doesn't always happen suggesting our immune systems are not working as well as they should.

We use terms such as "boosting our immune systems" loosely without really knowing what it means or how to achieve it. And a lot of this has to do with the fact that the immune system, as we have touched on, is immensely complex and has a huge number of variables.

Immune cell function

We have deliberately stressed the point that the immune system is cell-based; the intention is to convey the idea that, like so many other processes in the body, our ability to fight things such as infections and cancer, comes down to how optimally our cells are functioning. Our immune cells, just like any other cell, are subject to the vagaries of substrate availability, because they need energy to drive their processes. And just like any other cell this supply is potentially limited by IR.

The Renaut Equation

If we now bring IR into the equation it can be rewritten like this:

$$\text{Disease} + \text{Immune Response} (- \text{IR}) = \text{Outcome}$$

This is the Renaut Equation. It's not an equation in the strict mathematical sense, because the variables are not numbers. But If we now apply this to obesity and the very worrying statistics that show a much bigger risk of a whole range of serious conditions such as twelve different types of cancer, heart attacks, strokes, Alzheimer's Disease, osteo-arthritis and a large bunch of inflammatory conditions, then there are two clear possibilities. Either there is something in the fat-storage process itself that is promoting each disease, or there is something in the other variable, namely the immune response. Because these illnesses and diseases each have largely different causes (the cause of bowel cancer is different to the cause of breast cancer, for instance) it makes the first possibility extremely unlikely. And given that IR is the common factor in obesity, it's entirely logical and fair to point the finger at the immune response.

It explains in a logical way the underlying hypothesis in the Renaut Paradigm, which we'll learn about in chapter 9.

CHAPTER 8
THE DISEASES THAT ARE EVEN MORE COMMON IN OBESITY

Heart disease – Hypertension – Cerebrovascular disease – Cancer – Osteoarthritis – Obstructive sleep apnoea – GORD – Incontinence – Diabetes – Alzheimer's disease – Hypercholesterolaemia

---

Clinical studies on some common diseases tell us that they are even more common if you are either overweight or suffering from obesity.

With many diseases there are factors that initiate it and others that make it worse, and some of these factors are easy to identify. So, as an example we know without doubt smoking causes lung cancer – more than 95% of cases of lung cancer occur in smokers. In the small number of non-smokers who develop lung cancer it is more difficult to identify a cause and it may be that passive smoking is a contributor or possibly another cause altogether that we haven't yet discovered.

Similarly with osteoarthritis we know that this is due to degeneration in the biggest joints of the body in particular the hip, knee and shoulder as a result of wear and tear and injury. It's relatively easy to see a link between obesity and osteoarthritis simply because if you're carrying around more weight then there is going to be more wear and tear on the joints.

With other diseases, such as bowel cancer and breast cancer, we have identified some things that might possibly cause it, but in many people a particular cause cannot be identified or confirmed. In these diseases it is much more difficult to work out how obesity might be to blame, despite it being more common in this particular group.

As mentioned previously, we believe that it is in fact down to the immune system not working as well as it should; and we explain the reasoning behind this hypothesis. A lot of research is being done in most of these diseases and all we can really hope for is that at some point a cause will be identified. In the meantime, if you don't want to die prematurely, you are duty bound to try and reduce the risk where a risk factor like obesity has been identified.

Heart disease

Heart disease is a collection of conditions affecting the heart. It Includes diseases such as coronary artery disease, which is narrowing of the blood vessels that supply the heart muscle itself usually secondary to atherosclerosis or hardening of the arteries, and ischemic heart disease where there is an insufficient blood supply to the heart muscle which is secondary to coronary artery disease.

It also includes heart failure which is where the heart is unable to pump the blood around the body efficiently and there are number of reasons why this occurs. We also talk about valve disease – diseases of the heart valves in particular the mitral and aortic valves. A heart attack happens when the blood supply to the heart muscle is completely blocked and as a result a portion of the muscle dies. Sometimes this is sufficient to stop the heart beating resulting in a cardiac arrest and if this isn't treated with CPR within minutes then you die straight away. Even with CPR you can still die because the heart can't be restarted. If it is restarted, because the muscle dies, the patient often ends up with heart failure which can severely limit your ability to exercise or even climb the stairs.

The treatment of heart disease of course depends upon the underlying condition. Importantly most of these conditions are exacerbated by being overweight or by obesity so if you want to reduce your risk of these diseases and to live a happy, healthy, longer life then you need to address obesity itself.

Hypertension

Hypertension is the medical term for high blood pressure. The heart pumps blood around the body and in the process, develops a pressure gradient when the ventricle is contracting – this is about 120 mmHg and is known as the systolic pressure. Between contractions the pressure does not reduce to zero as there is elasticity in the blood vessels which initially expand and then contract to maintain the pressure gradient. This is known as the diastolic pressure and is about 80 mmHg.

There is a normal rage for both systolic and diastolic pressures in a healthy human. The normal range for systolic pressure is between 100 and 130 mmHg and for the diastolic this is between 60 and 90 mmHg. Minor variations don't really matter but if there are large variations over a period of time then this can have serious effects on the body.

The body has quite a simple feed-back system for maintaining and controlling normal blood pressure. It's in the form of some special cells called baroreceptors found in the carotid artery in the neck. They constantly monitor the pressure of blood in the artery – if it is low it activates the sympathetic nervous system which increases the pressure and if it is high the parasympathetic nervous system which lowers it.

We're not really certain what causes hypertension but certainly there are some significant risk factors such as smoking, being overweight or suffering from obesity. This is probably due to the extra work needed to simply pump the blood through the large amount of fat. In addition, because it is under cellular control, it is entirely possible that, in line with the Renaut Hypothesis, the baroreceptor cells are not functioning properly.

A chronically raised blood pressure, as previously discussed, can have dramatically harmful effects on the blood vessels themselves, in particular promoting hardening of the arteries through atherosclerosis which in itself can exacerbate hypertension. This in turn can increase the risk of conditions such as heart attacks and strokes.

Hypertension can also result in heart failure because the heart is simply unable to generate enough power to keep pumping the blood at the increased pressure. It can also lead to kidney failure with the result you need dialysis. Finally it affects the retina in the eye leading to loss of vision and eventually blindness.

Clearly if you have risk factors that are obvious then you are duty bound to deal with these in order to both avoid the need for pills to bring it into the normal range, or to avoid the long-term effects such as kidney failure and blindness. As being overweight or suffering from obesity are two of the most prominent risk factors then you can see a very compelling reason for dealing with this.

Cerebrovascular disease

Cerebrovascular disease is where the blood supply to a specific part of the brain is insufficient. The usual cause is either a narrowing of the blood vessels themselves, otherwise known as stenosis, or due to an actual blockage, or possibly due to a rupture of a blood vessel.

In all cases, the disruption of the blood supply results in a lack of oxygen getting to the part of the brain that the blood supply is feeding, and this will result in the brain cells (neurons) dying. This happens very quickly – within a matter of minutes and there is no ability for the brain to regenerate these dead neurons as there is with other cell types. And when neurons die, that part of the brain stops working. This is known as a cerebrovascular accident, or CVA for short, and in laymen's terms it is called a "stroke". It results in paralysis of the part of the body that is controlled by the corresponding area of the brain. If the affected part of the brain controls speech for example then the patient loses the ability to talk.

The usual cause of narrowing or stenosis of the blood vessels that feed the brain is the same process that causes heart attacks i.e. atherosclerosis. A great deal of research has been done and continues to be done into the cause of atherosclerosis and it is fair to say there is conflicting evidence about certain risk factors. Atherosclerosis involves damage to the vessel's very smooth lining resulting in inflammation and the development of a plaque which allows a thrombus or clot to stick to it. It can then become calcified resulting in a permanent narrowing of the blood vessel.

The narrowing itself can cause the blood flow to slow over a long period of time. But the other possible result is, because of its rough surface, a further clot or thrombus can form which then becomes dislodged and gets pushed along with the blood flow. The vessels get smaller the further away they are from the heart and at some point downstream the clot becomes lodged, completely blocking the flow of blood. The process of a thrombus forming and becoming dislodged, otherwise known as an embolus, is collectively known as a thrombo-embolic phenomenon and it tends to happen very quickly and with dramatic effect. The patient often becomes unconscious and dies within a matter of minutes.

Another type of cerebrovascular disease is the development of multiple small emboli affecting many areas of the brain over a long period of time leading to a gradual decline in brain function and leading to a form of dementia called multi-infarct dementia. An infarct means death of tissue.

A major risk factors for cerebrovascular disease is obesity. But there's also hyperlipidaemia (increased levels of bad fats in the blood), and type 2 diabetes, both of which are more common in patients who are either overweight or suffering from obesity. Because inflammation is once again a major part of the underlying pathology, you can see that if the inflammatory reaction is exaggerated, as in someone with a sub-optimally functioning immune system, then the potential for damage is greatly increased.

Whatever the mechanism it is clearly important that you should try to reduce your risk of developing the disease and the effects by dealing with obesity.

Cancer

Cancer in a nutshell is cell growth that is out of control. The word tumour comes from the Latin word tumor meaning swelling. Tumours are either benign or malignant, and a malignant tumour is synonymous with cancer. Cancers cells have the ability to lose their attachment to the primary tumour and to spread to other parts of the body where they grow into a secondary tumour otherwise known as a metastasis.

When a cancer metastasises, it does so either by spreading directly to nearby organs or via channels such as the blood vessels or more commonly the lymphatic vessels. When a tumour, either primary or secondary, gets to a size where it takes over the function of an organ, it will eventually kill the patient.

Our cells are programmed to die within a certain time period and to be replaced by new cells. This programmed cell death is known as apoptosis. However, if the cells don't die when they should then they continue to divide in a haphazard fashion. The older cells tend to develop genetic defects and then they function badly and produce proteins that are potentially harmful to the body.

The five commonest cancers that can metastasise and potentially kill the patient are, in order, lung, bowel, breast, prostate and kidney. So, these particular organs denote the site of the primary tumour. They can metastasise to any part of the body but the commonest places are to the lungs, liver and bones.

With some cancers, we know the cause. For instance, we know that in the vast majority of cases of lung cancer the patient is either a smoker or an ex-smoker who has smoked for many years. It does arise in a few patients who have not smoked and in these it is difficult to define a cause. In other types of cancer, the cause is less easy to identify.

With bowel cancer, for instance, we know that it is due to a series of gene defects, but we are not clear as to what actually causes the particular genes to become defective. And in fact, it may be a combination of agents such as a bacteria, virus or a chemical that has been released into the environment, or has found its way into our food chain.

Wherever the primary tumour has started, the treatment is the same – to get rid of it before it's had a chance to metastasise. With all of the five cancers mentioned above the initial treatment is surgical i.e. removal of the affected organ. Once a tumour has metastasised, unfortunately the chances of a cure are dramatically reduced. No amount of surgery on the primary tumour (beyond controlling the disease at the primary site) will alter the course of the disease. It is then a matter of relying on a combination of other therapies, in particular chemotherapy or radiotherapy, to try and deal with the metastatic disease.

Chemotherapy is the use of drugs that target and kill actively dividing cells such as cancer cells. Radiotherapy works in a similar way but instead uses ionizing radiation produced by radioactive isotopes to kill the cancer cells. But they also target dividing cells within normal healthy tissue and this explains the side effects such as sterility, diarrhoea and hair loss.

Clearly if we want to make advances with cancer then we need to concentrate on finding the causes and preventing it. Until that time, we have to rely on what we currently have, namely surgery for the primary disease and a combination of chemotherapy and radiotherapy for the secondary disease.

As far as obesity is concerned, we know that there are twelve different types of cancer, including breast and bowel, that are more common in these patients. But if we don't know what causes the cancer in the first place it's very difficult to work out how obesity is actually bringing about this increase.

One thing is quite certain: the immune system is crucial in determining the course and outcome of cancer in a particular individual and would explain partly why some patients live with their cancer to a ripe old age whilst others die relatively early. A quick glance down a microscope at a cancer that has been stained specifically for immune cells shows a host of specialised cells called tumour-infiltrating lymphocytes (TIL). They are there in an antigenic role (i.e. with the intention of trying to fight the cancer cells) but if the immune cells are not functioning optimally, as is possible in the patient with significant IR, then this might explain the increased incidence.

Yet another hypothesis is the role of autophagy which is described in chapter 1. Whatever the possible mechanisms, because we know that obesity is a risk factor, surely it's just common sense and logic to deal with it.

Osteoarthritis

Arthritis is inflammation of a joint and there are two main types, osteoarthritis and rheumatoid arthritis. The cause of the inflammation is completely different in the two conditions.

With rheumatoid arthritis, the inflammation is a type of autoimmune disease where the body's own immune system attacks and destroys the joints. We don't understand what starts it and therefore we can't cure it. It usually affects the small joints of the hands and the feet.

Osteoarthritis is inflammation of a joint caused by "wear and tear". It tends to affect the major joints of the body, i.e. the joints that typically have to do more work, so we are talking about the hips, knees, shoulders and the spine. We know that osteoarthritis is more common in patients who are overweight and suffering from obesity and this is almost certainly due to the fact that there is more weight to carry around in the form of fat.

In a normal healthy joint, there are usually two bones that articulate with each other. As an example, the knee joint is where the femur or thigh bone joins the tibia or shinbone. A joint between the bones simply wouldn't work, so the surfaces where they meet are covered by articular cartilage which is very smooth and is lubricated by fluid produced by the joint, called synovial fluid. This is effectively the body's lubrication oil.

With osteoarthritis, the articular cartilage is destroyed and this may happen because of the extra weight but also as a result of an injury that has happened in the past such as a fracture or a tear of the cartilage. This then exposes the underlying bone; and bone rubbing on bone makes the inflammation and pain worse.

The symptoms of osteoarthritis are limited movement due to stiffness but also pain, usually with activity. The treatment is simple pain relief with something like paracetamol but also a pain killer that specifically deals with the inflammation, so something like ibuprofen. However, in many patients this is no longer enough and if their mobility is badly affected to the point where they can no longer enjoy life, or even work, then a joint replacement needs to be considered.

Joint replacement surgery, such as a total hip replacement or a total knee replacement, replaces the whole joint with an artificial joint which is usually a combination of metal and plastic. This gives the patient back most of their mobility, but it never fully replaces the real thing and of course over time the artificial joint itself will wear out and after a few years may need to be replaced again.

Clearly the treatment of osteoarthritis needs to change from fixing things when they have gone wrong to preventing the problem in the first place and it's once again simple logic that if you're carrying around too much fat then you need to reduce it.

Obstructive sleep apnoea

Obstructive sleep apnoea, or OSA is a medical condition where you don't breathe enough during sleep. Apnoea means you actually stop breathing. It is due to a collapse of the upper airway and it's much more common if you are overweight or suffering from obesity.

An apnoea episode is defined as complete cessation of breathing for 10 seconds or longer. The patient typically is very tired during the day, and will wake up several times during the night with a gasping or choking sensation. There is loud snoring and frequent pauses in breathing during sleep, usually reported by a partner. There is fatigue and low energy due to the simple lack of sleep and the patient complains of an interrupted sleep pattern. OSA causes hypertension that doesn't respond to simple treatment, and it increases the risk of coronary artery disease and stroke, and increases the chances of premature death.

Individuals with OSA are rarely aware of any difficulty with their breathing even when they wake up. It is much more of a problem for the people close to them. Symptoms may have been present for years, and over time the individual tends to become used to the daytime sleepiness and fatigue that goes with sleep disturbance. Of course, if you sleep alone then you probably don't realise that you have a problem.

OSA is associated with obesity mainly through the increased amounts of soft tissues in the neck secondary to the excess fat. The treatment of OSA is mainly around identifying the risk factors and if these themselves can be reversed then the condition usually gets better by itself. Clearly if you are overweight or suffering from obesity then it goes without saying that this needs to be addressed as a priority.

Gastro-oesophageal reflux disease (GORD)

GORD is short for gastro-oesophageal reflux disease. In North America, it is known as GERD because they spell oesophagus incorrectly without the O. It is a very common condition affecting a large number of people and it is undoubtedly made worse by being overweight and by obesity.

The normal anatomy is fairly simple: after swallowing, food travels down the oesophagus or food pipe through the chest and as soon as it goes through the diaphragm, which is the muscular sheet between the chest and the abdomen, it opens up into the stomach. The stomach of course is a specific organ inside the abdomen.

The main function of the stomach is to hold the food for an hour or so and to break it up using contraction waves called peristalsis, before passing on to the next part of the gut called the duodenum. The stomach also has an enzyme that starts protein digestion. It also produces acid, making the contents of the stomach very acidic. The lining of the stomach can protect itself from these very acidic conditions but the rest of the gut can't and therefore damage can occur to the lining of these other parts if the stomach contents are allowed to find their way into these areas.

We're born with a valve between the oesophagus and the stomach which should keep the acid in the stomach and stops it going back up into the oesophagus. However, this valve sometimes becomes defective allowing acid to reflux and cause inflammation of the lining of the oesophagus, otherwise known as oesophagitis. The symptoms that result from this are called gastro-oesophagus reflux disease (GORD).

The main symptom is "heartburn", so called because it's located close to the heart. Typically it causes a burning feeling behind the sternum or breast plate and usually happens after eating as this is when the stomach is full and acid is being produced. It's also made worse by acidic or spicy foods and also by alcohol.

The reason why it is worse in obesity is probably because the abdomen has limited space and if this space is taken up by a significant amount of fat, this then increases the pressure and tends to force any gastric contents backwards making the GORD symptoms worse.

The treatment of GORD is usually something simple such as antacids which are alkali and which will effectively neutralise the acid in the stomach. More recently a class of drug called a protein pump inhibitor – or PPI – has been developed that stops acid being produced by the stomach.

Clearly however an important aspect of the disease is prevention, and if you are overweight or suffering from obesity then dealing with this problem will stand a good chance of relieving your symptoms so that you won't need any medication at all.

Incontinence

Incontinence happens when you can't control your bladder (urinary incontinence) or rectum (faecal incontinence) so you have accidents. It tends to be a lot more common in women, especially urinary incontinence, mainly because of the damage done to the pelvic floor when delivering a baby vaginally.

The pelvic floor is a series of muscles that are slung, like a hammock, from the inner aspect of the pelvis and are designed to keep the pelvic organs – the rectum, uterus and bladder – in their correct positions. When a baby passes through the middle compartment, the vagina, during child birth there is inevitably some damage to these muscles. As a result, generally later in life, the anterior and posterior compartments fall into the space occupied by the central compartment and, together with loss of power in the sphincter muscles, the patient experiences worsening incontinence.

The other thing that comes into play of course is what's happening above the pelvis from a pressure and mechanical point of view, based upon weight. It's obvious to see that if the abdomen is full of fat then this increases dramatically the pressure within the pelvis and pelvic floor, potentially making the incontinence a lot worse. It goes without saying that the first thing to do is to deal with your obesity. No amount of surgery is going to compensate for this, and in fact getting down to your BOW by applying the Nysteia Formula is your best way of avoiding this entirely.

Diabetes

The name diabetes comes from a Greek word meaning siphon, and is so called because all types of diabetes have one thing in common and that is polyuria or passing abnormally large volumes of urine. There are two main classes of diabetes. Firstly, diabetes insipidus and then the other main type which is diabetes mellitus.

Diabetes insipidus is rare compared to diabetes mellitus, which is the diabetes we all talk about and which is now very common and becoming more so. Diabetes mellitus is further divided into two types which we refer to as type 1 diabetes and type 2 diabetes. Type 2 diabetes is associated almost exclusively with obesity for reasons that we'll come on to shortly.

Diabetes was first recognised by Greek physicians who could tell the difference between the two types by tasting the urine. In fact, they used a small tasting spoon to sample the patient's urine. The urine in a patient with diabetes insipidus tasted as the name suggests – insipid. Whereas the urine in patients with diabetes mellitus (mellitus means honey) was sweet due to the sugar content.

Diabetes insipidus is due to a lack of a hormone called vasopressin, or antidiuretic hormone (ADH), which is produced by the pituitary gland in the brain and carefully regulates how much water the body needs by having a direct effect on the kidney. The usual cause is a benign tumour of the pituitary gland, preventing the secretion of the hormone into the blood.

The effect of vasopressin on the kidney is to reabsorb most of the water that is filtered by it and therefore a lack of this hormone results in the loss of body water through the urine. The end result is the passage of huge volumes of urine and there is a significant risk of becoming severely dehydrated in the process. In nearly all of us, this feedback loop works perfectly well and is the process by which the body regulates its own hydration. We also develop the sensation of thirst which tells us to drink more. The need to drink a minimum of eight glasses of water a day is complete nonsense – it just makes you run off to the toilet every hour, on the hour!

Diabetes mellitus is the body's failure to control the amount of glucose in the blood. Normally blood glucose sits within fairly strict levels i.e. 4.4 to 6.2 mmol/l. It can rise briefly to about 7.8 mmol/l in normal individuals after a meal, but is brought back down fairly quickly by insulin. If it rises above 11 mmol/l it fails to get filtered by the kidney and appears in the urine. This has an osmotic effect on the water in the kidney, effectively drawing it out and once again producing large volumes of urine.

The underlying problem with both types of diabetes mellitus is related to insulin. Insulin is the hormone secreted by the pancreas and is directly responsible for controlling blood glucose. In type 1 diabetes there is not enough insulin and in type 2 diabetes there is too much.

Type 1 diabetes is an auto-immune disease where the cells that produce insulin are destroyed by the patient's own immune system for reasons we don't understand, resulting in a failure of the pancreas to produce enough insulin in response to a rise in blood glucose.

The other type of diabetes mellitus is type 2 diabetes where there is an increased resistance to insulin, caused by too much insulin itself. There is a strong association with carrying too much fat: approximately 95% of type 2 diabetics are overweight or have obesity. The other 5% will have IR but they are genetically destined not to deposit fat the way the majority of us are. Pure logic says that if obesity was to cause IR, everyone who has IR must be fat. But as discussed, there's a group of diabetics (who by definition have significant IR) who don't have obesity, so it has to be the other way around – IR causes obesity. And this is proven by the fact that if you get rid of IR, by keeping insulin levels at zero for a significant part of the day, then obesity goes away.

Bizarrely this is completely opposite to what most doctors think, which goes a long way to explaining why we are failing to make any real headway in dealing with both obesity and diabetes. If they just understood that type 2 diabetes is caused by IR which is caused by producing too much insulin which, in turn, the body is forced to do in response to the mountain of carbohydrate that it's fed, then obesity and diabetes would go away. It's that simple!

The damage in both type 1 and type 2 diabetes is done not by the glucose being lost in the urine but by the effect that a chronically raised blood glucose has on certain organs. Excess blood glucose affects the small blood vessels causing narrowing and eventually gangrene; it affects the nerves resulting in numbness and paralysis; it affects the kidney producing kidney failure eventually requiring dialysis; and it affects the retina in the eye eventually causing blindness. The sum total is too horrific to contemplate and if people knew just half the story then common sense would surely prevail.

The treatment of type 1 diabetes is to replace insulin. This has to be given by injections because insulin is protein based and, like any protein, would get digested if it was taken orally. The treatment of type 2 diabetes is a bit more complicated. There are a number of different drugs that work by either helping the pancreas to produce more insulin or by reducing IR (or increasing IS). However, there comes a point where the IR becomes so great that these drugs no longer work and in these patients insulin is required to keep the blood sugar under control. Perversely this merely makes the IR worse because, as previously mentioned, IR is promoted by too much insulin.

A vital part of reducing IR is restricting the amount of carbohydrate in the diet. But just as important is reducing the frequency of food intake – this is precisely the reason for using intermittent fasting in the treatment of obesity and importantly the reason why it works. Not only does intermittent fasting deal with obesity through abolishing IR, but because type 2 diabetes is the next step, one would expect it to disappear. And in practical terms this is exactly what happens.

Alzheimer's disease

Alzheimer's disease is often referred to as simply Alzheimer's and is a chronic degeneration of the brain, otherwise called dementia. It accounts for 70% of cases of dementia, the other major cause being multi-infarct dementia (multiple small strokes – see above). We don't really know what causes it, but a significant part is believed to be genetic. Head injuries, depression and high blood pressure also appear to be risk factors. Importantly however, there is increasing evidence that being overweight and, in particular, having obesity are also risk factors.

The disease process is associated with the development of plaques and tangles in the brain. Early symptoms include short-term memory loss and problems with language, wandering off and getting lost, mood swings and generally not being able to able to look after yourself. Behavioural problems often follow including withdrawing from family and society. The gradual decline affects important body functions eventually leading to premature death.

As with many other diseases, it is difficult to identify a cause and effect, and its relationship with obesity may be nothing more than an association. It is entirely possible that it is related to IR directly affecting neurons, but the other possibility, in keeping with the Renaut Hypothesis, is an immune system that's not fully functional. Whatever the cause, because we know that there is an association with obesity, we once again have a responsibility in dealing with it in order to lessen our personal risk.

Hypercholesterolaemia

Hypercholesterolaemia means having increased levels of cholesterol in the blood. Cholesterol is a type of fat that is manufactured by the cells of the body and is an essential constituent of the cell wall. It is also a building block for important hormones such as corticosteroids. It is insoluble in water and therefore has to be transported in the blood in the form of lipoproteins of varying density: very low density, low density and high density lipoproteins (VLDL, LDL and HDL respectively). When you get your blood cholesterol measured it produces a figure that represents the total of these three things. But working out whether this is indicative of increasing your risk of heart attacks, for example, is not that simple because having a high HDL is in fact protective. Females are genetically determined to run higher HDL levels which might explain why, in general, they suffer less from ischaemic heart disease and strokes.

As previously mentioned, cholesterol is manufactured and metabolised by the billions of cells in our bodies and the amount produced, and therefore levels in the blood, are largely genetically determined. Contrary to popular belief, diet has minimal influence and in fact if you decrease your intake of dietary fats, with the intention of reducing your cholesterol level, then the cells just produce more.

Doctors get excited by cholesterol because there is some evidence that chronically elevated levels predispose to atherosclerosis which can then increase the risk of heart attacks and strokes. But as mentioned in previous sections, the process may not be as simple as this, and there is increasing evidence that inflammation in the artery wall may be an important underlying component. And this has added another level of complexity as to how best to manage it. The current conventional treatment is using statins but it's fair to say the jury is still out with regard to any true benefit. There are a number of clinical trials that have demonstrated conflicting results.

What is not in doubt is the association of hypercholesterolaemia with obesity and type 2 diabetes. In reality it is probably just this – an association. But because it is a manifestation of a cellular process it is relatively easy to see how, if your cells are functioning suboptimally, secondary to excessive IR, and in line with the Renaut Hypothesis and Paradigm, your cholesterol might be abnormally high. Irrespective of this potential, if you have a high cholesterol doesn't it make sense to deal with your obesity first? It might just save you from having to take yet another pill (which may or may not be beneficial) and with it the risk of a heart attack or stroke.

CHAPTER 9
WHY YOU WILL GET SICK AND DIE EARLY IF YOU HAVE OBESITY

The Renaut Paradigm

The Renaut Paradigm is: Unintended IR leading to metabolically-slow immune cells, disease initiation, disease progression and repair failure. The paradigm is based upon the Renaut Hypothesis. The definition of a paradigm is a pattern or a model. A hypothesis is an idea.

In line with the hypothesis, IR affects immune cells and is an unintended consequence of a normal survival mechanism that has been carried to an extreme, leading to an increased incidence of disease. As discussed in previous chapters, there was a survival advantage in primitive man having the ability to conserve his stored energy substrates – glycogen in the case of glucose and adipose tissue in the case of fatty acids. For this to happen it would require the body to have a mechanism for slowing down its cellular metabolism. In effect a mini-hibernation.

Insulin receptors exist to control how much glucose enters the cell, so one of the ways of regulating a cell's metabolism is to limit the amount of substrate. Down-regulating the receptor will do exactly this and it happens when there is too much insulin which then leads to IR. An excess of insulin happens in the fed state. It's a simple and effective way of regulating the metabolism of individual cells, the sum of which is our total energy expenditure.

CHAPTER 9 | 87

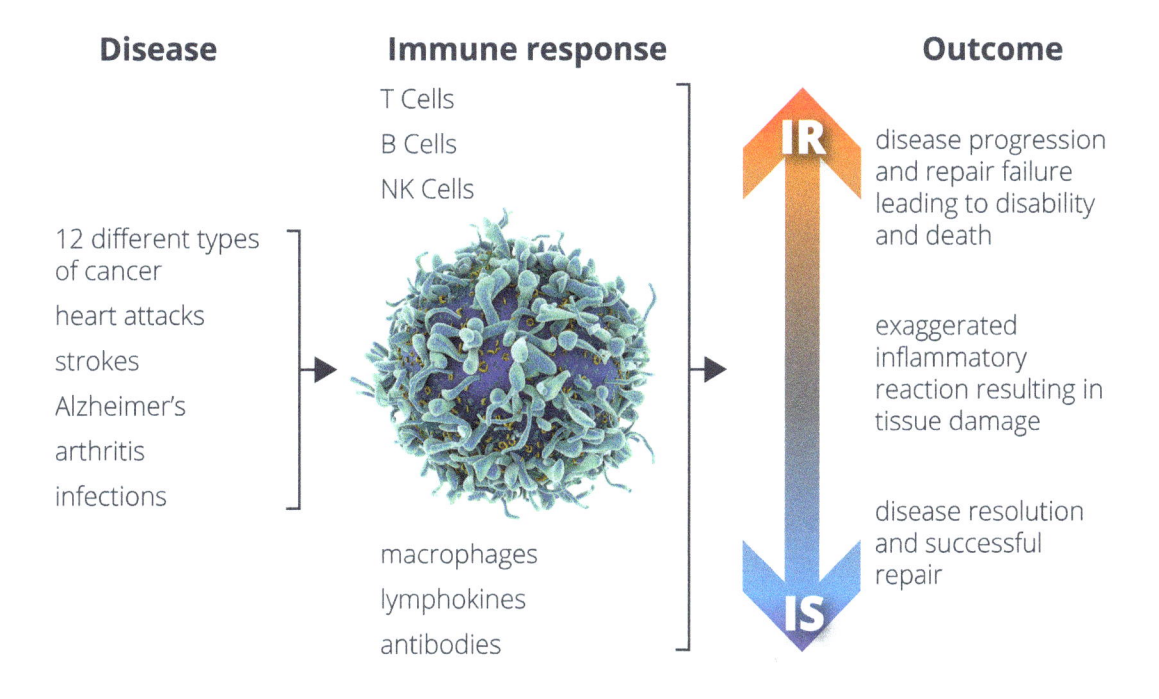

The Renaut Paradigm
Insulin resistance and the immune response

Disease

12 different types of cancer
heart attacks
strokes
Alzheimer's
arthritis
infections

Immune response

T Cells
B Cells
NK Cells

macrophages
lymphokines
antibodies

Outcome

IR — disease progression and repair failure leading to disability and death

exaggerated inflammatory reaction resulting in tissue damage

disease resolution and successful repair

IS

Figure 11. *The Renaut Paradigm - insulin resistance and the immune response*

When the food supply ran out insulin secretion dropped and the cells regained their IS allowing glucose back into the cell and boosting metabolism. This put the body back into a state of readiness that allowed him to search for more food. All cells have insulin receptors and are therefore subject to the variable state of IR versus IS. However, primitive man never had the luxury of a constant food supply, and the change from one state to the other was relatively small and occurred over short periods of time. Any potentially detrimental effects were minimal. Now let's fast forward to our current eating habits where food is always in abundance. The storage facility and the mini-hibernation facility still exist, but if we are taking in the typical western diet of refined carbohydrate at frequent intervals, then we either never develop, or we lose over time the IS that our cells and bodies evolved to function with. It's a sure-fire bet that you'll have some IR unless you are applying the Nysteia Formula (or something very similar). Under these circumstances, your immune cells, which are subject to IR just like any other type of cell, are constantly in a hypometabolic state simply because glucose can't get in.

When this is applied to the Renaut Equation, as described in chapter 7, then it would explain why you have a greater risk of getting diseases such as heart attacks, strokes and cancer if you have too much subcutaneous and visceral fat. It's not the obesity that causes the disease. It's IR leading to suppression of the immune system. Figure 11 shows how this happens. It would also explain why your appetite disappears during illness – it's your body's way of forcing itself back into full IS, thereby ensuring that the immune system is working to its maximum capacity.

We would stress that this is merely a hypothesis. The really good thing however is that an intervention and a clinical trial are not required to prove this hypothesis. The intervention has already been done in the form of introducing refined carbohydrate into the western diet without, alarmingly, any evidence as to its benefit or safety. In fact, quite the opposite – there is now very good evidence that it has had a profoundly detrimental effect on our health.

In summary, IR slows metabolism – that's what it's meant to do. The aim should be to allow all cells to operate with optimal function and to re-establish IS by applying the Nysteia Formula. It's the only way you'll achieve it and in the process you're simply allowing the human body to function the way that it has evolved to survive. You will also be at your BOF and your BOW and your disease risk will be very low.

CHAPTER 10
WHAT YOUR ULTIMATE GOAL SHOULD BE

Insulin sensitivity – Biological optimum function (BOF) – Biological optimum weight (BOW)

Biological optimum function (BOF) and biological optimum weight (BOW) are two concepts that we've developed within Nysteia. They relate to having minimal IR or conversely full IS. The ultimate aim is to achieve and maintain BOF and this equates to optimal cellular function. This can only happen by allowing your cells to enjoy full IS. As a happy coincidence you will also be at your BOW.

Insulin sensitivity

This is the inverse of IR. As discussed in previous chapters, we believe IR is a normal survival mechanism that has evolved to ensure that we conserve our stored energy substrates when in the fed state, and determines how hard your cells are working by limiting the uptake of glucose. Which is all well and good up to a point. But if taken beyond this point, as in the continuously fed state, then it has significant unintended consequences. It promotes the conversion of carbohydrate to fat, it slows down your cells and, through its effect on your immune cells, puts you at greater risk of severe disease. As a result, you become fat, experience physical and mental tiredness and you are at significantly increased risk of being sick.

The way to regain IS is easy – just reverse the process that produced IR. The best method we know for doing this is by using the Nysteia Formula.

Biological optimum function (BOF)

This is where all the cells in your body are metabolising and functioning with maximum efficiency. Whatever their specific role – be it neurons transmitting electrical impulses, red blood cells carrying oxygen, gut cells digesting food or baroreceptor cells maintaining normal blood pressure – they are doing it without restriction. And this is of course vital because the thousands of biological processes and chemical reactions that are occurring constantly in our bodies, without us even having to think about them, have evolved over hundreds of thousands of years to ensure that we survive. So we need to make sure they are allowed to do exactly this, because if we don't our chances of survival are lessened. And that's exactly what we see in practical terms.

A cell's metabolism can be slowed by restricting the supply of substrate that provides energy – just in the same way that the engine in your car can is controlled by how much fuel you give it via the accelerator. The way this is done in the human body is far more sophisticated than in a car. The two main substrates are glucose and fatty acids. The secondary ones are amino acids, ketone bodies and alcohol.

The supply of glucose to the cell is never in doubt even in starvation because of gluconeogenesis but, as part of our evolution, the body has developed a clever method of slowing down the entry of glucose *into* the cell which was needed in primitive man when the body was in the fed state so as to preserve food stores and conserve energy substrate.

Insulin itself does this – by way of a beautifully designed feedback loop. Lots of food, especially carbohydrate, results in a large insulin response which in turn, over time, down-regulates the insulin receptor stopping glucose from getting into the cell. And very conveniently the same hormone switches off lipolysis, therefore limiting the availability of fat as well. Overall body metabolism (BMR) falls and we slow down.

In primitive man, if food was in short supply, insulin would be at low levels and as a result, the cells would get back their IS allowing glucose back into the cell, boosting metabolism and putting him into a state of readiness to allow him to get his next meal. We have deliberately designed the Nysteia Formula to copy these conditions; but the really good news is that your food supply, if you're in a developed country, is never in doubt.

You can now see how IR dictates cellular metabolism by regulating how much glucose enters the cell. And your BOF, which equates to optimal mental and physical wellbeing, is the sum total of your cells' metabolism. In practical terms it also equates to your BOW and a PBF of about 10% - just enough fat reserves to stop muscle being used up as energy but not so much that it slows our efforts at doing day to day tasks.

The other very important thing to note when you reach your BOF is that you will stay there, along with your BOW, with very little input, apart from continuing with the Nysteia Formula indefinitely. And this is because your body will be in equilibrium. It will tell your brain exactly how much energy substrate is required so that your food intake matches expenditure.

On days when you might take in more than you need, for instance if you go to a dinner party and eat and drink more than usual – and you instinctively know when this happens – you will make up for it over the next few days. You will only run into trouble of course if you make a habit of it.

Biological optimum weight (BOW)

Getting down to your BOW and staying there needn't be the ultimate aim. You will get there though as a happy consequence of having maximal IS and having BOF. Happy because having more fat than you need is a huge source of unhappiness in many of us. It is that weight that you will automatically reach when you follow the Nysteia Formula.

If you allow your body to simply perform its normal homeostatic mechanisms, especially the ones dealing with nutrition and energy substrates, as intended, then it will achieve and maintain an optimum PBF which in most of us is between 10 and 12% of total body weight. This obviously equates to a particular weight that is different for all of us, based upon the composition of our other body parts, e.g. how big our muscles and bones are.

BOW is therefore not an absolute figure. Nor does it equate to a strict BMI. There's no doubt your BOW will be within the healthy BMI range of 18 – 25. That said, it's not really necessary to measure your BMI regularly as it involves measuring your weight and doing the calculation. A much easier way of reaching your BOW, without the risk of getting obsessed by it, is simply to apply the Nysteia Formula – you will automatically arrive at your BOW. You will know when it happens because you will wake up one morning, look in the mirror and shout "YES!".

As far as staying at your BOW is concerned this is equally straight forward – you simply continue with the Nysteia Formula indefinitely. If you go back to the things that got you into trouble in the first place, well then the inevitable will happen. The really great thing about achieving your BOW is that psychologically you feel a new person and you can go out and buy yourself a new wardrobe of clothes which you will never have to throw away. Fashions do a full circle and they will still fit in 20 years' time!

CHAPTER 11

THE NYSTEIA FORMULA – THE THREE THINGS YOU NEED TO DO TO CHANGE YOUR LIFE

Intermittent fasting – Cardiovascular exercise – Mediterranean-type cuisine

The Nysteia Formula is the practical application of Nysteia's philosophy. Nysteia's philosophy is to achieve physical and mental wellbeing by making some simple yet significant changes to your life-style. Central to this is dealing with obesity and in the process getting down to your biological optimum weight (BOW), getting rid of insulin resistance (IR), regaining insulin sensitivity (IS), and allowing you to achieve and maintain biological optimum function (BOF).

Having read all of the information in the preceding chapters, you will now have a basic, but sound understanding, of how your body handles food and importantly how you get obesity and may become sick in the process.

The Nysteia Formula is effectively a quick start guide that will tell you how to arrive at your BOF and BOW, how to abolish IR and regain maximal IS. It allows you to get started here and now.

When it comes to how food causes obesity there are three things to consider: the **AMOUNT** of food you eat which is important, the **TYPE** of food you eat which is very important and finally **WHEN** you eat it which is absolutely critical. The Nysteia Formula tackles all three factors.

It's important to understand that the Nysteia Formula it is not a diet – but it does require you to do things differently in order to bring about change. In the words of Albert Einstein: the definition of insanity is doing the same things over and over again and expecting different results. If you **don't** want to change, the Nysteia Formula isn't for you. If you **do** want to change then the Nysteia Formula is all you need.

Intermittent fasting

In the Nysteia Formula the 24-hour day is divided into an 18-hour fasting window and a 6-hour feeding window. This has been done for a very good reason – an 18 hour fast is easy to do for most people and importantly it allows the body to use its stored fat as an energy substrate when glucose is in limited supply. The 6-hour feeding window is similarly an adequate period of time for most people to get in their daily calories (2000-2500 Calories) without the pressure to do so in a shorter time period.

Most individuals will stop eating at about 7pm and then will fast when sleeping until the following morning. It is then a simple matter of continuing with the fast for another 6 – 8 hours. For practical purposes this means going without breakfast and to have lunch at about 1pm. During this period, you will certainly get hungry and this can be helped by regular cups of black coffee, green tea or simply tap water, none of which contain any calories and therefore do nothing to your insulin.

The other important aspect of intermittent fasting is its regularity. Because humans are creatures of habit, once you are into the routine of an 18-hour fasting window and 6-hour feeding window it becomes much easier to do. And in fact, after a couple of weeks it becomes so routine that you just treat it as a normal way of life.

Fig 12 is a guide showing you when you should and shouldn't eat.

Recommended 24-hour intermittent fasting schedule

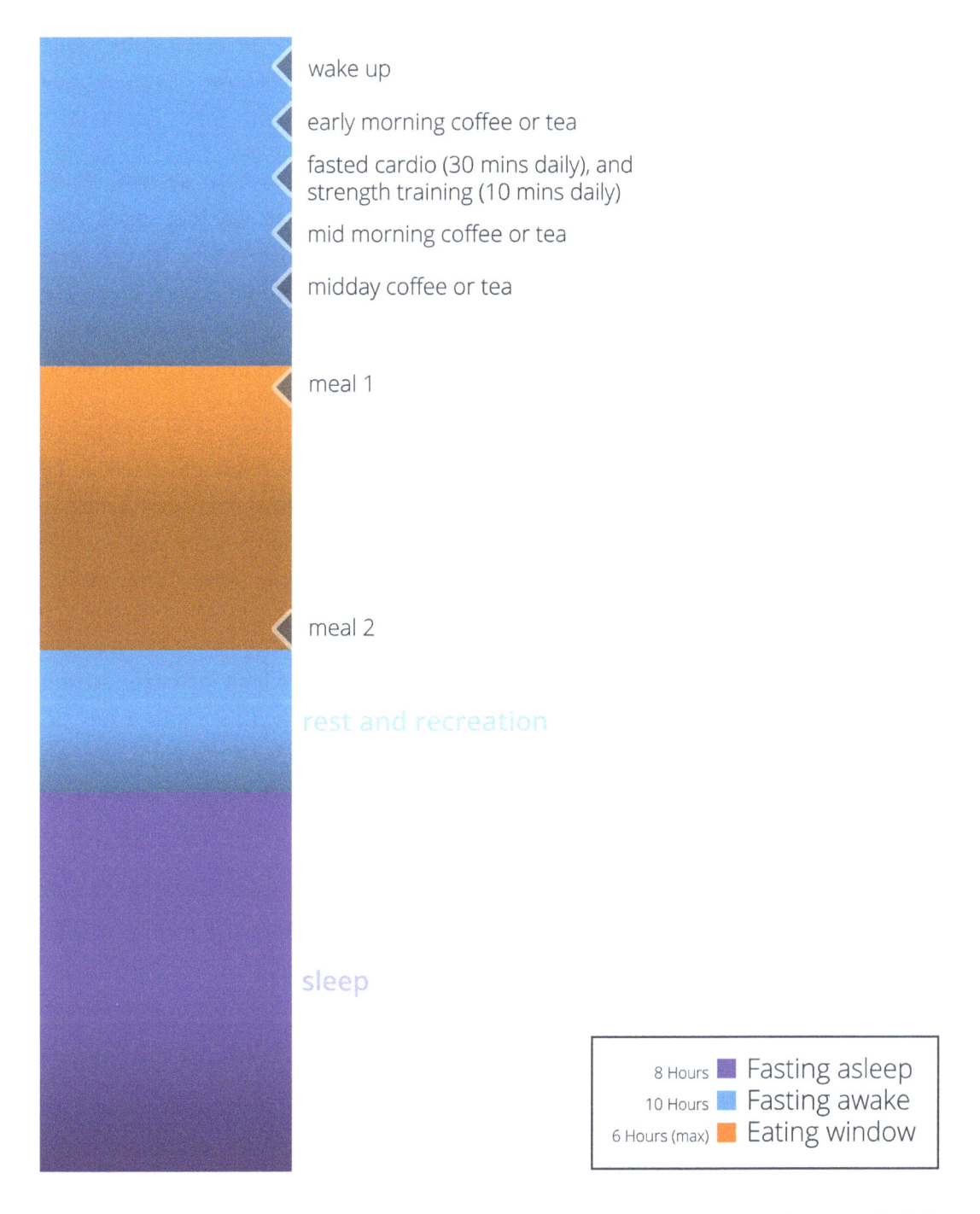

- wake up
- early morning coffee or tea
- fasted cardio (30 mins daily), and strength training (10 mins daily)
- mid morning coffee or tea
- midday coffee or tea
- meal 1
- meal 2
- rest and recreation
- sleep

8 Hours	■	Fasting asleep
10 Hours	■	Fasting awake
6 Hours (max)	■	Eating window

Figure 12. *Recommended 24-hour intermittent fasting schedule*

Cardiovascular exercise

Cardiovascular exercise is an essential part of the Nysteia Formula and is absolutely vital, by definition, to achieving and maintaining optimal health and fitness. It works in three ways: it is an evolutionary survival mechanism and, when done in the fasted state, it gets rid of your glycogen stores forcing the body into lipolysis (the breakdown of stored body fat); it also gives your heart muscle a workout.

It is so called because of the effect that it has on your cardiovascular system, which is your heart and blood vessels. It is defined as any physical activity that raises your heart rate. Regular exercise has been shown to have a very positive effect on general health and lifespan. And of course the opposite is true as you would expect. If you are overweight or already suffering from obesity then it's only natural that you will find any form of exercise difficult, even walking. But the good news is that even a brisk walk to start with will increase your heart rate.

You must understand however that, despite what you've always been told, exercise by itself will not get the weight off and that's because by itself it doesn't affect IR which is the underlying problem in obesity. This can only be done by changing the way you eat and from a practical perspective the thing that works in the long-term is intermittent fasting and limiting refined carbohydrates.

As time goes on you will steadily lose weight and your exercise limit increases so you can walk faster and faster and then you will break into a jog and then into a run. So, the answer is to start gently and to build up over time. The important thing is to push yourself a little bit further each and every day so that after half an hour you can feel your pulse increase, you are sweating and you are out of breath – that's how you know you've done some good.

If walking and running aren't for you it's important that you find something that is, such as cycling, swimming or going to the gym. Ideally it should be done first thing in the morning whilst you are still fasting – don't worry, your body has plenty of reserves and that's exactly what you want it to use.

The energy you need for exercise is obtained from your reserves which are your liver and muscle glycogen stores that have been topped up from the day before. If you're trying to lose weight then it's important to deplete these early in the day and this will happen with a good bout of exercise. This ensures that you get into fat burning for a good 6 hours before you start eating again. And it's important that you do it every day for at least 30 minutes – no more excuses!

Mediterranean-type cuisine

Mediterranean-type cuisine is a concept we have developed within Nysteia and is really quite specific. It is essentially a mix of all three macronutrients – carbohydrate, fat and protein – in moderate quantities.

One of the most important bits of Mediterranean-type cuisine is the exclusion of sugar, anything with added sugar, processed food (which almost certainly contains some added sugar) and refined carbohydrate. Also, anything labelled as "low fat" – the fat has been taken out and sugar added to make it taste better. If you eat any of these it will raise your insulin and if this is done often enough and with big enough meals, you will definitely develop significant IR which of course will promote obesity.

There are 28 countries that have a Mediterranean coastline i.e. a connection with the Mediterranean Sea, and they all have their own cuisines. The thing that connects all of these countries is the abundant use of fresh ingredients and this is something that we think is absolutely vital when it comes to the food we eat.

The other main reason for calling it Mediterranean-type cuisine is that it does not exclude other types of cuisine that are just as healthy such as Japanese cuisine and the food you find in other countries in south east Asia.

APPENDIX

What's included in Mediterranean-type cuisine

Below is a list of foods and drinks that we consider are included in the idea of Mediterranean-type cuisine, and also the difference between what you should eat for weight loss and weight maintenance as described in chapter 2. It is purely a guide. A large part of this journey is working out for yourself what is healthy and what is not so healthy and a lot of this comes down to common sense.

What you can eat for weight loss

• Broccoli	• Nuts
• Beans and lentils	• Red meat
• Avocados	• Fish (Salmon, tuna, White fish)
• Carrots	• Chicken (any poultry)
• Zucchini	• Eggs
• Eggplant	• Tomatoes
• Onions & spring onion	• Cheese
• Garlic	• Olives
• Cauliflower	• Peanut butter
• Lettuce	• Milk & cream
• Asian veg (e.g. pak choy or bok choy)	• Yoghurt
• Capsicum	• Butter
• Cucumber	• Orange (1 a day)
• Radishes	

What you can eat for weight maintenance

Everything in the category above, plus *(in moderation)*	
• Rice	• Pasta
• Sweet potato	• Pumpkin
• Bananas	• Any fruit (1 or 2 small daily portions only in addition to the orange)

What you can drink

• Water	• Black coffee
• Green tea	• Black tea - only if you find either black coffee or green tea unacceptable (a dash of milk in any beverage is acceptable if it means that without the milk you would not be able to drink it)
• A glass or two of good quality red or white wine with your evening meal. Alternatively, a single shot of spirit such as whiskey or vodka.	

What you can't eat

• Sugar	• Anything processed
• Anything with added sugar (essentially anything out of a packet or a jar)	• Anything "low fat" (sugar will have been added)
• Bread	• Crisps
• Cookies, cakes & muffins	• Potato
• Cereals	• Ice cream
• Candy	• Chocolate

What you can't drink

• Soda (including no-sugar or reduced-sugar equivalents)	• Mixers e.g. tonic water and ginger ale
• Cordial	• Beer
• Protein smoothies	• Iced tea (unless you've prepared it yourself with no added sugar)
• Fruit juices	
• Fruit smoothies	

Abbreviations and their definitions

BOF   **Biological Optimum Function** – the state of the body's cells, and therefore the body as a whole, when IR is completely abolished and full IS is regained.

BOW   **Biological Optimum Weight** – the weight you will automatically descend to and maintain when you have BOF. Equates to a PBF of about 10% and a BMI of 20.

BMI   **Body Mass Index** – a practical way of measuring obesity. Equates to weight (in Kg) divided by height (in metres) squared e.g. a person who weighs 70kg and is 175cm tall will have a BMI of 70 ÷ (1.75 x 1.75) = 23.

BMR   **Basal Metabolic Rate** – the energy required by the sum total of your cells when in the resting state. Generally fixed and determined by the relative proportions of IR and IS.

CAL   **Calorie** (Kcal or a thousand calories). A Calorie (capital C) is a thousand calories (small c). A calorie is specifically a unit of heat energy and is the amount of energy required to raise the temperature of 1ml of water through 1deg Celsius. 1 calorie = 4.2 joules.

CNS   **Central Nervous System** – collectively the brain and spinal cord.

CO   **Cardiac Output** – the volume of blood, measured in litres per minute, put out by the heart. CO = HR x SV. Can double or even triple with cardiovascular exercise.

GI   **Glycaemic Index** – a relative value given to a food type, relating to how rapidly the blood sugar rises after its breakdown and absorption in the gut. Indirectly determines the insulin response.

GORD   **Gastro-Oesophageal Reflux Disease** – a collection of symptoms and signs related to the reflux of acid from the stomach into the oesophagus.

HR   **Heart Rate** – the number of beats of the heart per minute. Increases with cardiovascular exercise.

IF   **Intermittent Fasting** – eating all of your food within a dedicated period and having no food for the remainder of the 24-hour period. Does not require calorie-counting and is definitely not starvation.

IR   **Insulin Resistance** – a cellular state preventing glucose from entering the cell in response to chronically elevated insulin levels.

IS	**Insulin Sensitivity** – a cellular state allowing glucose to enter the cell unrestricted. The inverse of IR.
KJ	**Kilojoule** – a thousand joules. A joule is the SI unit of energy and is equivalent to the amount of energy exerted when a force of one newton is applied over a displacement of one meter. 1 calorie = 4.2 joules.
NF	**The Nysteia Formula** – the practical application of Nysteia's philosophy: intermittent fasting, cardiovascular exercise and Mediterranean-type cuisine.
OSA	**Obstructive Sleep Apnoea** – a medical condition where the individual stops breathing for extended periods during sleep.
PBF	**Percentage Body Fat** – the amount of subcutaneous and visceral fat within the body expressed as a proportion of the total body weight.
SV	**Stroke Volume** – the volume of blood (in mls) put out by the heart with each beat. Increases with cardiovascular exercise.
TDEE	**Total Daily Energy Expenditure** – the total amount of energy used by the cells of the body in a day. Equates to BMR plus the energy required for physical exertion and processes such as digestion.

FAQ

Why am I fat?

Am I fat because I have bad genes?

No. We all come from the same gene pool, and they are doing exactly what they are supposed to do. And that is to convert excess carbohydrate into fat and then to store it.

Am I fat because I have a slow metabolism?

No. Your metabolism (BMR) will certainly be slow if you have significant insulin resistance (IR) and this relates to your chronically elevated insulin levels as a result of consuming large amounts of refined carbohydrate at regular intervals. IR dictates whether glucose goes into the cell for immediate use or gets converted to triglycerides and then gets stored as fat. So it's IR that causes your obesity and at the same time gives you a low BMR.

Am I fat because I don't do enough exercise?

No. Exercise by itself will not get rid of IR which can only be done through changing the way you eat.

Am I fat because I'm eating wrongly?

Yes. In particular you are eating too much refined carbohydrate too often. This results in chronically elevated insulin levels leading to IR.

If I don't change the way I eat will I always be fat?

Yes. Einstein's definition of insanity is doing the same things over and over again and expecting different results. It's really not that difficult.

Will those clever scientists invent a pill that will get rid of my fat allowing me to eat whatever I like?

No. Billions of dollars are wasted on trying to find a cure when it's entirely preventable in the first place. Research into the causes of obesity and trying to find a cure only exists for the benefit of the people who work in it.

The food that I eat

Should I be eating fresh meat, fish, vegetables, nuts and dairy?

Yes. In fact fresh wholefoods are all you need to eat. The takeaway pizza is quite possibly the worst thing to afflict humanity.

Should I avoid food out of a packet?

Yes. It's been processed to a variable degree and almost certainly has added sugar. And it generally tastes nothing like the real thing. Don't be lazy – learn to prepare it yourself from fresh ingredients.

Should I avoid "low fat" foods?

Yes. The fat has been taken out and sugar added. Fat does not make you fat because it doesn't influence insulin levels that much. Refined carbohydrate makes you fat through the development of IR. Animal fats were demonised by the US government 50 years ago and we've been paying the price ever since. There is very little evidence, if any, that demonstrates a risk with heart disease.

Are there certain foods that will boost my metabolism?

No. Quite the opposite in fact. The huge amount of refined carbohydrate that you have been chowing down over the years has led to significant IR, which stops glucose getting into cells and decreases metabolism. The only thing that will boost it is getting rid of IR which means cutting out carbs.

Is fresh food more expensive than fast food?

No. You're just using that as an excuse for your laziness. If you shop around you will find fresh food that in fact is cheaper than fast food and is a lot more nutritious.

Is it acceptable to have someone else prepare and cook my food every day?

No. If your health and the food that you eat are not your No1 priority then your priorities are seriously out of whack.

Are coffee shops dangerous places?

Yes. The counters are stacked full of refined carbohydrate. A black coffee is healthy – it's the huge portion of chocolate gateaux that goes with it that's killing you – literally. They need to be avoided at all costs.

Do the cereal and soft drink companies and fast food chains give a damn about my welfare?

No. The only thing they care about is taking your money.

Does my body have a requirement for any amount of sugar in my food?

No. It has no requirement whatsoever. Anyone who tells you otherwise is lying to you.

Can I eat fruit?

Yes. But only in small amounts. Fruit contains a natural sugar called fructose which contributes to IR and which the cells will use as an energy substrate instead of fatty acids.

Can I drink alcohol?

Yes. In limited quantities – a glass or two of wine with dinner. Like fructose it is used by the cell as an energy substrate. However, good quality wine helps you to see eating as a celebration and not just a way of relieving your boredom – psychologically it's very good for you.

If I eat lots of protein will my muscles get big and will the girls fancy me?

No. Your body only requires about 0.8g of protein per kg of body weight per day. So for a 70kg person that's about 60g. Anything more than that gets flushed down the toilet or gets converted to fat making your obesity worse. It's a really stupid thing to do.

Your body, health and disease

If I skip breakfast will I collapse in a big heap?

No. What do you suppose primitive man had for breakfast - rice crispies? Your body has a very sophisticated mechanism called gluconeogenesis that ensures your blood sugar is kept within a very strict range even after weeks of starvation. The only way you can become hypoglycaemic is if Dr Renaut injects you with insulin.

Am I constantly exhausted because of stress?

No. Your exhaustion is due to mental and physical fatigue secondary to IR which is slowing the entry of glucose into your brain and muscle cells respectively. And you're stressed, anxious and depressed because you don't like the way you look and feel. The priority is to eliminate IR by using the Nysteia Formula – which will then boost your BMR, allowing you to function optimally. As a result your weight loss and feel-good factor will make your stress evaporate and you will be a new person.

If I have obesity is there a good chance I will develop some nasty disease that will result in a painful, horrible, slow and early death?

Yes. You have a significantly increased risk of getting 12 different types of cancer, heart attacks, strokes, Alzheimer's and a whole host of inflammatory conditions. And if you develop type 2 diabetes, secondary to IR, you are at risk of blindness, kidney failure and gangrene. If you get gangrene, a surgeon like Dr Renaut will come along and chop your leg off.

Do I need to take vitamin supplements and the like?

No. There is no single macronutrient nor micronutrient that is completely depleted within an 18 hour fast so you are never going to run into deficiencies, with the caveat that you are eating fresh and nutritious food within your 6-hour feeding window. You might as well save yourself the time and just throw your money down the toilet because that's where it eventually ends up. Better still, if you want to give away your money simply post it to Dr Renaut and he will look after it for you.

Exercise

Do I need to exercise every day?

Yes. It needs to be cardiovascular exercise which is any activity that raises your heart rate for 30 minutes, ideally in the fasted state. You cannot use the excuse that your knees won't allow it. Your knees hurt because you are carrying the equivalent of a 30kg sack of potatoes around every minute of the waking day.

Is it acceptable to use the excuse that I'm too busy to exercise when in fact I spend all my time on social media?

No. Let's face it – you're not fooling anyone.

Can I exercise the weight off?

No. Exercise in isolation does not address IR. It has to be done as part of the Nysteia Formula.

Is exercise harder to do because I'm fat?

Yes. But not necessarily because of the extra work required to carry around the extra fat. It has a lot more to do with the fact that your muscle cells have IR which stops the glucose getting in, leading to early fatigue. When you get rid of IR by using the Nysteia Formula, your exercise regime suddenly becomes a whole lot easier and more enjoyable. Inform your personal trainer of this snippet of information because the only thing they know is how to thrash you to within an inch of your life. And how to take your money.

The Nysteia Formula

Is it just another fad diet?

No. It's not a diet at all – it is a way of life and a method of eating and is something you do for the rest of your life. The Greeks did it 3000 years ago, so hardly a fad.

Is IF the same as ketosis?

No. Ketosis is the generation of significant quantities of ketone bodies – three separate compounds derived from triglycerides in the liver after about three days of starvation. Intermittent fasting (IF) encourages lipolysis which is completely different and is the breakdown of triglycerides into fatty acids which are then used by the cell as an energy substrate in their own right. The term 'ketogenic diet' is used by people such as personal trainers, exercise physiologists and celebrity chefs who clearly have no understanding of how the human body works.

Is IF the only biologically proven method of sustainable weight loss?

Yes. Because it's the only way we know that completely abolishes IR.

Can I eat anything in the fasting window?

No. By definition. But you can drink unlimited amounts of black coffee, green tea and water, as they do not raise your insulin.

Can I eat what I like in the eating window?

No. But realistically the only thing you need to eliminate is refined carbohydrate. See: What's included in Mediterranean-type cuisine.

Do I need to count calories?

No. It is a complete waste of time and the calorie-restricted diet has been shown to fail every time anyway. For it to work you would need to know what your calories-out figure is and this is impossible to calculate. If you're doing the NF your sense of satiety will automatically limit your daily intake within the 6-hour feeding window. Regaining IS ensures your TDEE is boosted well beyond your intake, putting you into a calorie deficit without you even having to think about it.

Do I have a personal responsibility to deal with my obesity, having been given all the information I need in The User's Manual For Your Body?

Yes. It is not the responsibility of the people around you to pick up the pieces. You have run out of excuses.

Printed in Australia
AUHW010653171019
318712AU00001B/1